# universal beauty

## The Miss Universe
## Guide to Beauty

FOREWORD BY DONALD J. TRUMP

# universal beauty

## The Miss Universe Guide to Beauty

cara birnbaum

RUTLEDGE HILL PRESS®
Nashville, Tennessee
A Division of Thomas Nelson Publishers
www.ThomasNelson.com

Published by Rutledge Hill Press, a Division of Thomas Nelson, Inc., P.O. Box 141000, Nashville, Tennessee 37214.

Rutledge Hill Press books may be purchased in bulk for educational, business, fundraising, or sales promotional use. For information, please e-mail SpecialMarkets@ThomasNelson.com.

The views and opinions expressed in this book are those of the individuals interviewed and do not necessarily reflect the views or opinions of Donald Trump, Miss Universe L.P., LLLP, or any company related to Miss Universe L.P., LLLP ("Miss Universe Organization"). The Miss Universe Organization does not make any representations, warranties, or assurances as to the accuracy, currency, or completeness of the information provided and shall not be liable for any damages or injury resulting from readers' reliance on any information provided. The information contained in this book is for general informational purposes only, and is not intended as health or medical advice. Readers should not rely on this information to determine a diagnosis or course of treatment and should always consult with a physician before making any changes in medication or lifestyle as a result of any information contained in this book.

Photograph credits appear on page 209, which constitutes a continuation of this copyright page.

The trademarks displayed herein are the property of their respective owners.

Illustrator:  Annie-France Giroud (represented by American Artist Reps, Inc.)

Creative Directors:  Jessica Feder and Frank Szelwach

Interior Designers:  Bill Chiaravalle, DeAnna Pierce, Mark Mickel, Brand Navigation, LLC.

**Library of Congress Cataloging-in-Publication Data**

Birnbaum, Cara.

  Universal beauty : the Miss Universe guide to beauty / Cara Birnbaum.

      p. cm.

  Includes index.

  ISBN 1-4016-0229-0 (hardcover)

  1.  Miss Universe Pageant. 2.  Beauty, Personal. 3.  Feminine beauty (Aesthetics)  I. Title.

  HQ1219.B57 2006

  646.7'2--dc22

                                        2005030910


*Printed in the United States of America*

06  07  08  09  10  —  5  4  3  2  1

*Though we travel the world over to find the beautiful,*

*we must carry it with us or we find it not.*

—Ralph Waldo Emerson

To all the titleholders who have represented,

and continue to represent,

the Miss Universe Organization so very graciously,

thank you for being beautiful, inside and out!

# CONTENTS

# ACKNOWLEDGMENTS

The Miss Universe contest is a beautiful collaboration uniting men and women across the globe, from camera crew to government officials, to the stunning women who compete for the crown. So it's fitting that this book has also been a true team effort. While it's impossible to individually thank everyone involved, I'd like to mention a handful.

First, the Miss Universe Organization thanks the titleholders, former and current, whose beauty, grace, charisma, hard work, and philanthropy set an example for women around the world, year after year. These are strong women with enviable looks and lives. They are lawyers, politicians, heads of companies, actresses, models, mothers, wives, and so much more. Many of them endured long interviews and shared beauty secrets that their husbands don't even know. Just a few notables: Natalie Glebova revealed how to walk in high heels, Jennifer Hawkins disclosed why she rarely suffers from blemishes, Amelia Vega expounded upon the merits of raw egg whites, Brook Lee and Margaret Gardiner told us about their remarkably low-maintenance primp routines, Porntip "Bui" Nakhirunkanok Simon and Martha Vasconcellos detailed why they'll never go without sunscreen, Angela Visser sent adorable pictures of her daughter, Wendy Fitzwilliam outlined her trick for keeping skin hydrated during air travel, Maritza Sayalero waxed poetic about lipstick, and Yvonne Agneta-Ryding mused about her long walks in the woods.

Thank you to our wise and wonderful group of experts, who contributed a wealth of information about keeping the body gorgeous and healthy from head to toe. Among them, makeup artists B.J. Gillian from CoverGirl and Linda Rondinella-Osgood, dermatologist Cheryl Thellman-Karcher, hairstylist John Barrett, hair colorist William Howe, Reebok Sports Club fitness trainers Clayton James and Robert Sidbury, dentists Allyson K. Hurley and Radford Y. Goto, the Miss Universe Organization's style gurus Billie Causieestko and David Profeta, and manicurist Jin Soon Choi. I was amazed to find out about the Miss Universe Pageant's large and devoted base of followers, including its number one fan and historian, William Prendiz, who was an invaluable resource.

This book would be nothing without the photographers and artists who translated pages of amazing advice into stunning pictures and illustrations. The Miss Universe Organization's phenomenal creative directors, Jessica Feder and Frank Szelwach, worked tirelessly, during long nights and weekends, to orchestrate this book's production. (I suspect Frank knows more than he ever cared to about hair removal and proper blush placement.) Finally, thanks to my husband, Jake Harmon, for always making me smile when I was on deadline. After all, as Sylvia Hitchcock Carson (Miss Universe 1967) explained so well, smiling is the best beauty secret of all.

—Cara Birnbaum

Beautiful women are one of the great joys in life—maybe the greatest joy, as far as I'm concerned. While I've written a lot about the art of the deal, I believe beauty is also an art. Like any other art form, it should be celebrated and appreciated.

The television ratings for the Miss Universe Pageant, which I've owned since 1996, indicate that the world is very interested in beautiful women. This is not a big surprise to me, but it's nice to know I've got plenty of company. That's one reason I've decided to present *Universal Beauty: The Miss Universe Guide to Beauty* for worldwide consumption.

As with all of my endeavors, I have decided that only the best will do. So in the following pages you will be presented with the best as it pertains to beauty. The Miss Universe Pageant has become the United Nations of glamour, and this book reflects the global aspect and influence of this most coveted of beauty competitions.

The first Miss Universe Pageant was in 1952. It was one of the first showcases for true diversity, and it has served to shape and widen today's notion of beauty. It is now at the top—the icon of all pageants. I don't produce anything less than the best or the most exclusive, and this pageant reflects that standard. So does this book.

In the following pages, you will find a pictorial history of the Miss Universe Pageant, a glimpse of behind-the-scenes events at the competition, insider beauty tips, and step-by-step directions for applying professional beauty secrets in your everyday life. Every day is an event, whether or not you're Miss Universe, and this book will help you achieve the look that makes Miss Universe the most sought-after title in the world of beauty.

Enjoy, learn, and indulge in the art of beauty. Beauty is very much a treasure. And it's a treasure you can develop and enhance by reading *Universal Beauty: The Miss Universe Guide to Beauty.*

—Donald J. Trump

# universal beauty

## The Miss Universe Guide to Beauty

PART 1

# pageant beauty

# the miss universe pageant: then and now

The Miss Universe competition is known as a showcase for the world's most glamorous, poised, stunning women. So it's hard to believe that the pageant started in 1952 as a promotional event for Catalina Swimwear. Twenty-nine women, dressed in one-piece white bathing suits, vied for the crown that day in Long Beach, California. During the weeks leading up to the big competition, the contestants had traveled first to New York City, where some of them tasted hot dogs for the first time. They watched a Yankees game, stayed at the top-end Plaza Hotel, then boarded a Pan Am jet bound for the West Coast. At the pageant Armi Kuusela, an eighteen-year-old high school student from Finland, walked off with a Romanoff crown that had once belonged to a Russian czar. It was made of no fewer than 1,529 diamonds with a combined weight of 300 carats.

Today's Miss Universe crown is no slouch either. Valued at approximately $250,000, the coveted Mikimoto headpiece contains 800 diamonds and 120 pearls—and comes with an armored case to withstand the rigors and security hazards of constant airplane travel. The number of contestants who vie for this crown every year has skyrocketed to over eighty. And those white one-piece swimsuits that started it all look pretty tame compared to the white bikinis and stilettos contestants parade in these days. But one thing hasn't changed during the past half century. Year after year, Miss Universe continues to remind us of the glorious beauty of diversity.

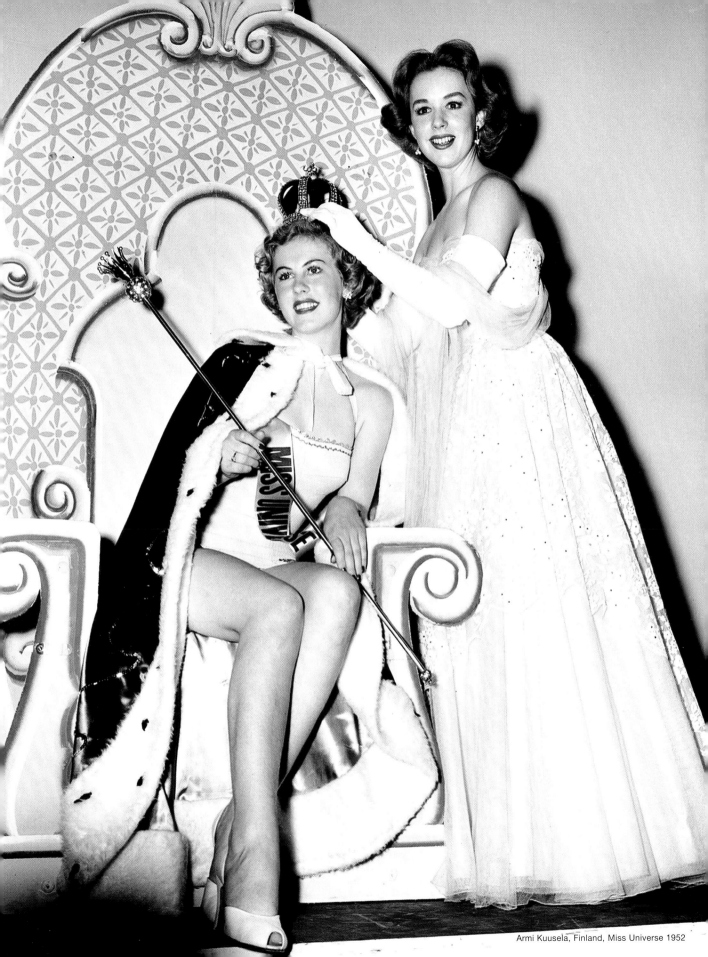

Armi Kuusela, Finland, Miss Universe 1952

# beauty through the years

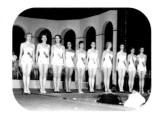

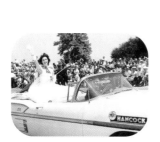

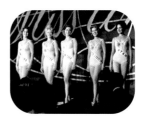

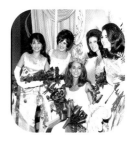

## 1952
Catalina Swimwear creates and sponsors the first Miss Universe and Miss USA competitions as concurrent events in Long Beach, California. They feature twenty-nine contestants and are not televised.

## 1957
Peruvian-born Gladys Zender becomes the first Latin American Miss Universe, then appears on *The Ed Sullivan Show.*

## 1960
The Miss Universe competition moves to Miami Beach, Florida, and makes its television debut on CBS.

## 1967
Perhaps inspired by the hit musical *Hair,* the Miss Universe competition drops its ban on hairpieces.

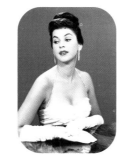

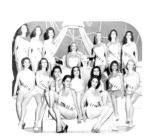

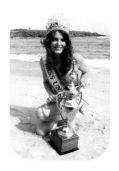

## 1961
Young, up-and-coming TV personality Johnny Carson hosts the pageant.

## 1958
Luz Marina Zuluaga wins the title, and the Colombian government awards her a ten-bedroom mansion. Three postage stamps, three national songs, and a Max Factor lipstick are created in her honor.

## 1956
Contestants are no longer allowed to marry before or during the year of their reign.

## 1972
The competition begins to telecast from exotic locations around the world. Puerto Rico is the first host outside the continental United States.

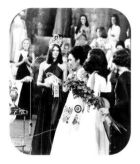

## 1973
Philippines First Lady Imelda Marcos calls in the military to seed monsoon clouds in an effort to diffuse a storm that threatens to cancel the Miss Universe competition.

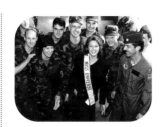

## 1990
The first contestant representing the USSR participates in the Miss Universe competition.

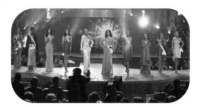

## 2001
The Miss Universe and Miss USA competitions celebrate their fiftieth anniversaries.

## 2003
NBC becomes co-owner of the Miss Universe Organization, and the Miss Universe Pageant makes its NBC debut live from Panama City, Panama.

## 1984
The Miss Universe Pageant returns to Miami after a twelve-year absence.

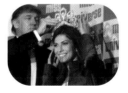

## 2002
Oxana Fedorova is stripped of the Miss Universe 2002 title for failure to carry out her obligations. First runner-up Justine Pasek of Panama is crowned Miss Universe 2002 by pageant owner Donald J. Trump at one of the largest press conferences ever held at Trump Tower.

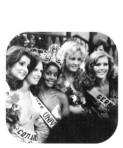

## 1977
Janelle Commissiong (Trinidad & Tobago) becomes the first black woman to win the Miss Universe title.

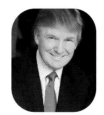

## 1996
Donald J. Trump purchases the Miss Universe Organization.

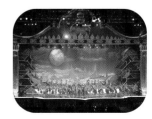

## 2005
The Miss Universe Pageant is distributed to a record 170 countries and territories.

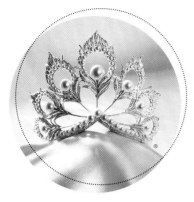

# miss universe titleholders

● ● ● ● ●

| 1952 | 1953 | 1954 | 1955 | 1956 | 1957 |
|---|---|---|---|---|---|
|  |  | 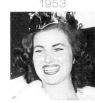 |  |  |  |
| **Armi Kuusela** Finland | **Christiane Martel** France | **Miriam Stevenson** USA | **Hillevi Rombin** Sweden | **Carol Morris** USA | **Gladys Zender** Peru |

| 1958 | 1959 | 1960 | 1961 | 1962 | 1963 |
|---|---|---|---|---|---|
| 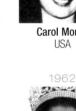 |  | 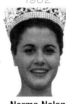 |  | 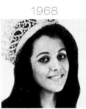 | 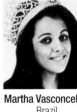 |
| **Luz Marina Zuluaga** Colombia | **Akiko Kojima** Japan | **Linda Bement** USA | **Marlene Schmidt** Germany | **Norma Nolan** Argentina | **Ieda Maria Vargas** Brazil |

| 1964 | 1965 | 1966 | 1967 | 1968 | 1969 |
|---|---|---|---|---|---|
|  |  |  |  |  |  |
| **Corinna Tsopei** Greece | **Apasra Hongsakula** Thailand | **Margareta Arvidsson** Sweden | **Sylvia Hitchcock** USA | **Martha Vasconcellos** Brazil | **Gloria Diaz** Philippines |

| 1970 | 1971 | 1972 | 1973 | 1974 | 1975 |
|---|---|---|---|---|---|
| 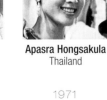 |  | 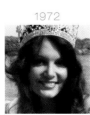 |  |  |  |
| **Marisol Malaret** Puerto Rico | **Georgina Rizk** Lebanon | **Kerry Anne Wells** Australia | **Margarita Moran** Philippines | **Amparo Munoz** Spain | **Anne Marie Pohtamo** Finland |

| 1976 | 1977 | 1978 | 1979 | 1980 | 1981 |
|---|---|---|---|---|---|
|  | 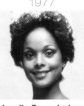 |  | 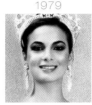 |  |  |
| **Rina Messinger** Israel | **Janelle Commissiong** Trinidad & Tobago | **Margaret Gardiner** South Africa | **Maritza Sayalero** Venezuela | **Shawn Weatherly** USA | **Irene Saez** Venezuela |

| 1982 | 1983 | 1984 | 1985 | 1986 | 1987 |
|---|---|---|---|---|---|
|  | 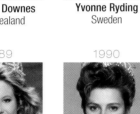 |  |  |  | 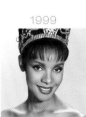 |
| **Karen Baldwin** Canada | **Lorraine Downes** New Zealand | **Yvonne Ryding** Sweden | **Deborah Carthy-Deu** Puerto Rico | **Barbara Palacios Teyde** Venezuela | **Cecilia Bolocco** Chile |

| 1988 | 1989 | 1990 | 1991 | 1992 | 1993 |
|---|---|---|---|---|---|
|  | 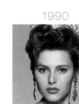 |  |  |  | 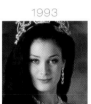 |
| **Porntip Nakhirunkanok** Thailand | **Angela Visser** Holland | **Mona Grudt** Norway | **Lupita Jones** Mexico | **Michelle McLean** Namibia | **Dayanara Torres** Puerto Rico |

| 1994 | 1995 | 1996 | 1997 | 1998 | 1999 |
|---|---|---|---|---|---|
|  | 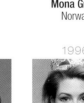 |  |  |  |  |
| **Sushmita Sen** India | **Chelsi Smith** USA | **Alicia Machado** Venezuela | **Brook Lee** USA | **Wendy Fitzwilliam** Trinidad & Tobago | **Mpule Kwelagobe** Botswana |

| 2000 | 2001 | 2002 | 2003 | 2004 | 2005 |
|---|---|---|---|---|---|
|  |  |  |  |  | |
| **Lara Dutta** India | **Denise M. Quiñones August** Puerto Rico | **Justine Pasek** Panama | **Amelia Vega** Dominican Republic | **Jennifer Hawkins** Australia | **Natalie Glebova** Canada |

# beauty behind the scenes

If you're vying to be named the most stunning woman on the planet, there may be no tougher place to do it than Bangkok in May. Morning temperatures soar into the makeup-melting nineties. Come noon, the sun is strong enough to turn the most enviable complexion blotchy and burned within minutes. It all makes for one steamy, pore-clogging, urban rain forest.

So when Thailand's bustling metropolis hosted the Miss Universe contest in May 2005, beauty products and tools took center stage—behind the scenes, anyway. While eighty-one of the most alluring women in the world prepared to greet a television audience of one billion, their dressing rooms filled with clouds of hair spray, compacts of CoverGirl makeup flew like Frisbees, and flat irons glided over unruly frizz at mach speed. By the time the young women took the stage for the opening dance number, they were ready for their close-ups. Magdalene Walcott's (Trinidad & Tobago) caramel complexion looked poreless and radiant. Ieva Kokorevica's (Latvia) tresses tumbled over her shoulders in buttery waves. And though Canada's Natalie Glebova had spent the past three weeks waking up for 3 AM photo shoots, often after attending late-night parties with the rest of her fellow ambassadors of beauty, she had little trouble wooing the judges, who awarded her the coveted Mikimoto crown. "I spotted her from the beginning—there was just this extra glow, energy, and a real charisma," says model Heidi Albertsen, who sat on the 2005 judges' panel.

But let's face it, Heidi knows as well as anyone that, when it comes to seducing the spotlight, a team of experts with a few tricks up their sleeves certainly doesn't hurt. We ducked into the dressing rooms to spy on how the planet's premiere beauties prep for the camera.

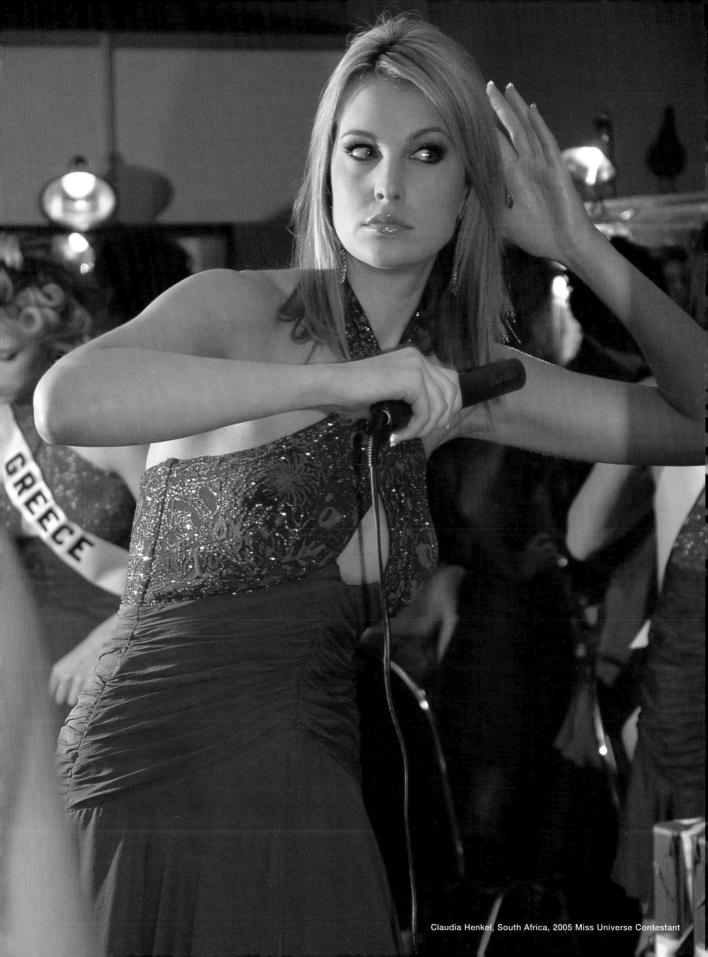

Claudia Henkel, South Africa, 2005 Miss Universe Contestant

# pores, shine, and other dirty words

In a perfect world, pageant skin is a smooth, flawless canvas. In other words, it shouldn't betray a hint of oil, acne, or even obvious pores—even when the forecast calls for 100 degrees and 100 percent humidity as it did in Bangkok in 2005. Linda Rondinella-Osgood, the hair and makeup coordinator for Miss Universe, reveals her backstage recipe for complexion perfection.

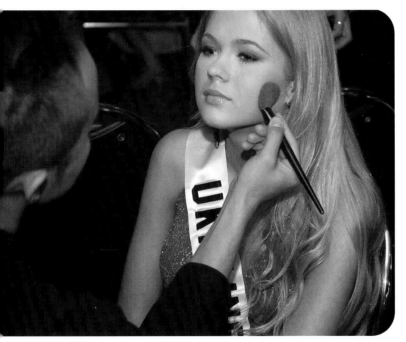

Juliya Chernyshova, Ukraine, 2005 Miss Universe Contestant

**Come clean.** "I always make sure to start with a freshly washed face," says Rondinella-Osgood, who follows with an allover swab of astringent to make sure every pore is clear of grime and product residue.

**Moisturize.** You want to moisturize—but only where necessary. Because makeup will look chalky and uneven if applied over flaky spots, smooth rough patches with a drop of oil-free lotion—then leave the rest of the face alone so it doesn't look greasy later.

**Choose the right base.**
Ensuring that skin looks as flawless during the last five minutes of the pageant as it did during the first requires foundation specifically designed to stand up to hot lights and sweaty conditions—in other words, professional-grade formulas. "I use Gerda Spillman bases," says Rondinella-Osgood. "Their colors match virtually any skin tone out there, which is really what you need for a show that's as diverse as Miss Universe. The consistency isn't too thick or too thin, and it covers anything that ails you."

**Apply it right.** Backstage, where makeup artists may touch more than twenty faces in two hours, foundation goes on with a clean, dry sponge, which doesn't spread bacteria the way fingertips can. It's then smoothed over the entire face and blended down into the neck.

**Disguise the extras.** Those not trained in makeup artistry should probably stick to concealers that match our skin, but professionals such as Rondinella-Osgood use an orange-toned formula to neutralize dark, bluish under-eye circles and a tan one to mask red marks from pimples and clusters of veins. "Then I blend, blend, blend!" she says.

**Lock in the job.** The big secret to preventing a makeup meltdown when the competition heats up: Rather than simply dusting translucent loose powder over the face, use a large puff to actually *press* it into the skin.

**Don't forget to blush.** A light pop of blush is another must for keeping the face from disappearing under stage lights. Before smiling their way onstage, Miss Universe contestants grin for the makeup artist, which reveals the apples of their cheeks. A swirl of powder blush is brushed over each (cherry red for dark skin, pale pink for fair skin, and raspberry for olive skin), then blended up and out toward the temples.

# made in the shade

The global beauties competing for the crown may be blessed with exceptionally good bone structure—but more often than not, they've had a little outside help. Stage and screen makeup artists frequently use powder a shade darker than the foundation shade to reshape the jaw-line, nose, and eyes.

**Define the cheekbones.** Makeup artists have the girls suck in their cheeks and shade just above the hollows.

**Downplay a long nose.** Brush contouring powder down the center.

**Narrow a wide nose.** Shade either side of it.

**Use caution.** Most experts say facial contouring is far too risky for real life where stripes of dark makeup will only end up looking like dirt.

## universal truth

To keep skin from looking washed out under bright lights, Rondinella-Osgood uses foundation that's one shade darker than the skin.

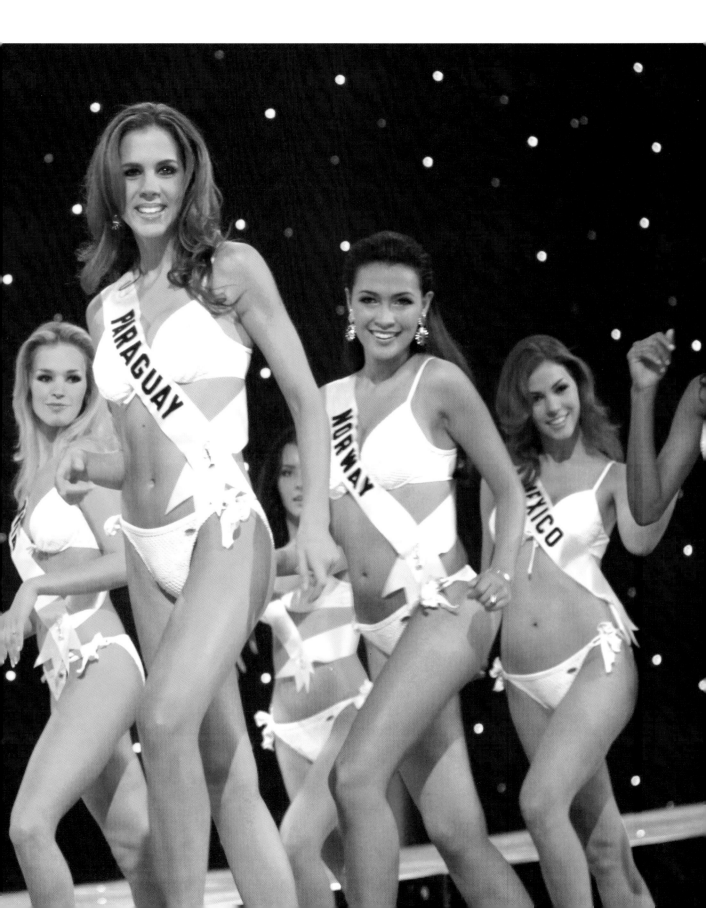

By the time you see them on TV, the Miss Universe contestants have spent a grueling three weeks dancing through long rehearsals, shuttling to parties, and coping with serious jet lag. So how can they possibly look so radiant the day of the show? "I sleep between events—and sometimes *at* events," said one recent contestant from Trinidad & Tobago.

Those with no time to snooze can at least reach for a makeup bag.

### Light up with a luminizer.
This cream or powder with the slightest hint of shimmer can make a tired face look refreshed and awake. Makeup artists dot luminizing powder along the tops of the cheekbones and along the brow bones. Just be warned: Obvious shimmer or glimmer can be disastrous and distracting on TV. If anyone else can tell you're wearing luminizer, you've put on too much.

### Swab on under-eye highlighter.
To make the eyes look brighter and more alert, Rondinella-Osgood brushes powder one shade lighter than the foundation under the eyes, then blends it up to the lids. Some makeup artists even highlight lower lashlines with white pencil.

### Add a fake fringe.
Backstage pros rarely let a Miss Universe hopeful go without adding false eyelashes. While strips tend to weigh down the lids, individual clusters of lashes placed near the outer corners perk up the eyes instantly. Once the glue is dry, the entire fringe is crimped with a lash curler.

### Amp up your lashes.
Mascara is an absolute must—three coats is usually the minimum before showtime. To pile on the goop without disturbing the rest of the face, Rondinella-Osgood has girls close their eyes, then places a tissue just underneath the lashes and flat against the cheek. "This way, I can knock myself out applying mascara on top of the lashes, curling them upwards with the brush."

# the better bod

When asked how many crunches, squats, and treadmill miles they slogged through during the final few weeks before the big day, most of the girls we polled in Bangkok in 2005 admitted the answer was zero. We sleuthed around backstage to uncover how they make up for those lost days in the gym.

Spotted: fake bake. Fiona Hefti (Switzerland) sported a golden glow that she later admitted was faux. "This was my first time using self-tanner—I put it on two days ago," she said. Smart girl: When you're pale and pasty, even the slightest bit of excess flesh can look more obvious.

Spotted: shimmer lotion. Luminizing lotion made an encore performance as Chananporn Rosjan (Thailand) slathered the Body Shop's Cranberry Shimmer Body Lotion all over her legs and arms. A bit of shine (again, the operative word is "bit") can make calf, arm, and abdominal muscles look more toned and defined.

Spotted: double-stick tape. Nearly all the girls used it—perhaps most commonly beneath their bikini bottoms to keep them from riding up the rear.

Spotted: body makeup. To hide bruises and small clusters of veins, the pros rolled out the heavy-duty cover-up. Rondinella-Osgood's favorite line of concealing creams for body blemishes: Joe Blasco. She dots it on the imperfection, blends well, then sets it with loose powder.

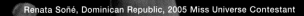
Renata Soñé, Dominican Republic, 2005 Miss Universe Contestant

# countdown to gorgeous

Working one's way to the Miss Universe crown has always been an art form. And nowhere is this more evident than backstage, where an extra flick of mascara or a properly angled curling iron can help make or break a girl's chances. Here, a look back at some of the best moments in pre-pageant primping.

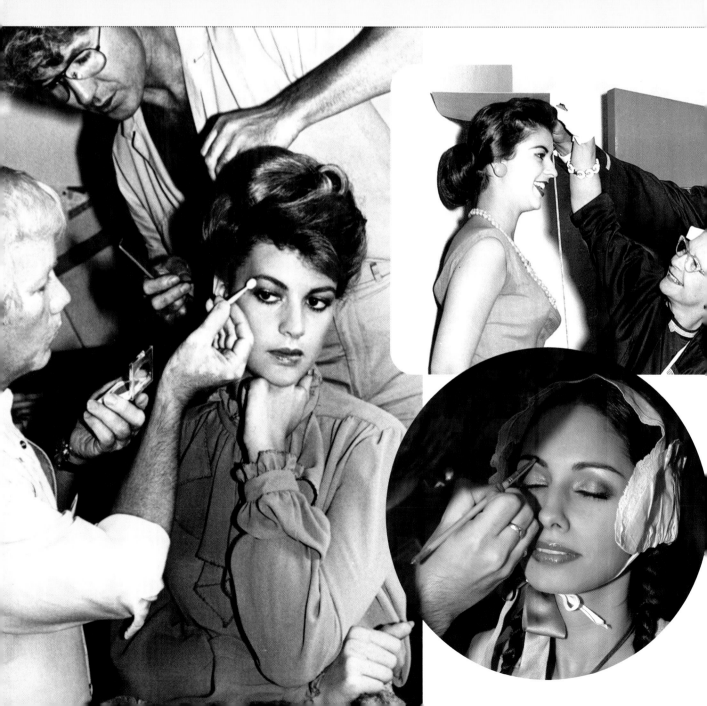

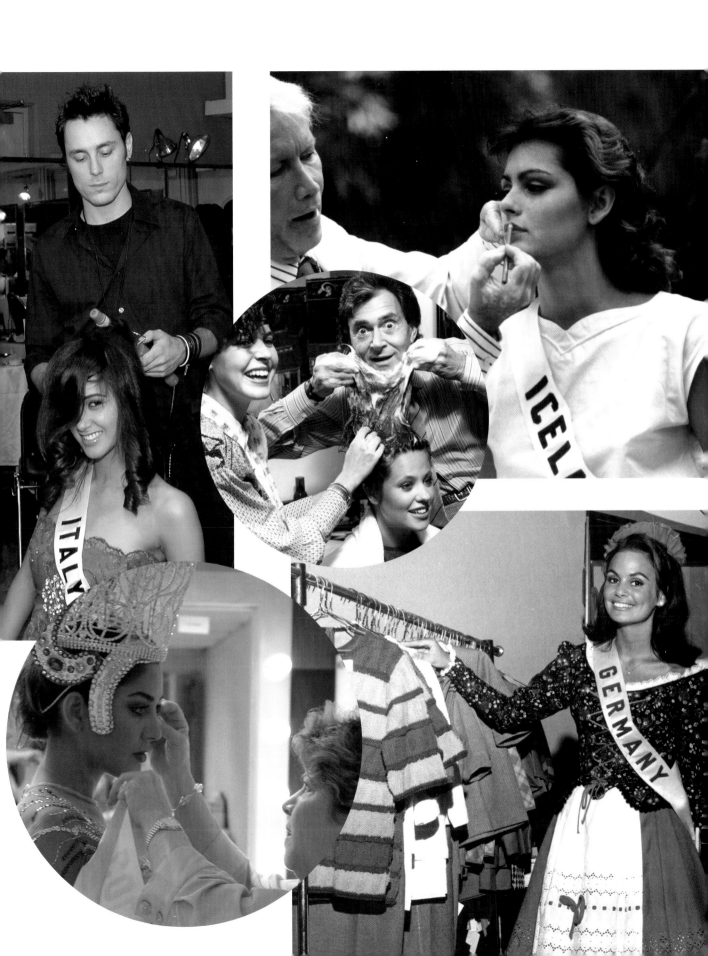

# finishing touches

Miss Universe is about celebrating diversity—not turning international beauties into identical Barbie dolls. So makeup artists examine contestants as individuals—enhancing the very best features for the most flattering, natural look. To keep the face from looking clownish or overdone, the pros focus on only one area of the face (typically either the lips or the eyes) and use minimal color on the rest.

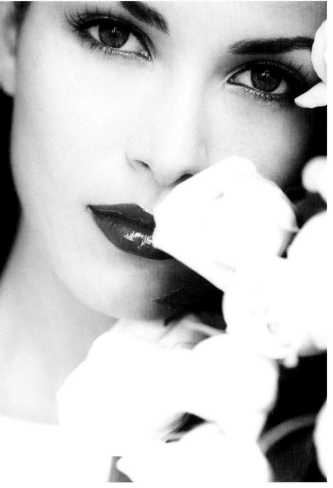

Justine Pasek, Panama, Miss Universe 2002

## gloss alert

If too much glimmer spells *danger* on the face, it's downright deadly on the lips. Spotlights and cameras magnify shine, turning it into a distraction for the judges—especially if the gloss ends up sinking below the lips onto the chin. "You'll look like you're drooling!" warns Linda Rondinella-Osgood. Even worse, with all that dancing and head swinging, it's only a matter of time before the hair sticks to the mouth, dragging the shiny goop onto one cheek—not a good look. The pros advise choosing light, non-goopy formulas—and only applying a light film at a time.

## the stay-put pout

The beauty queen's trick for keeping lipstick in its place:

1. Smile, then outline the mouth with a lip pencil.

2. Use that pencil to fill in the lips to prevent ring-around-the-mouth later.

3. Top with a matching lipstick, then with a touch of non-sticky gloss.

4. For extra staying power, press loose powder onto the lips over the liner and under the lipstick.

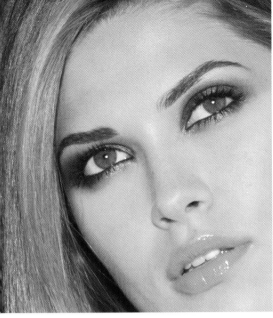

Justine Pasek, Panama, Miss Universe 2002

## eye spy

Makeup artists backstage have huge palettes of eye shadow at their disposal. But regardless of which colors they choose, placement usually follows a standard formula.

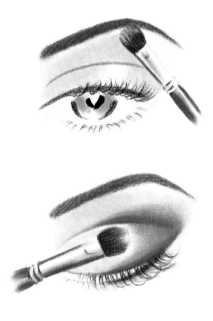

1. Select two coordinating shades—one lighter and one darker.

2. Dampen the eye shadow brush slightly, dip it in the lighter shade, and apply a light wash of the color all over the lids and up to the brow bone.

3. Dip the brush into the darker shade, and draw a fuzzy line from the center of the lash line (where the pupil is) to the outer corner of the eye, and then up to the center of the crease. (The shape should look like a letter *V* turned on one end.)

4. Blend the entire eye area to erase any obvious lines.

## brow-wow!

Piles of eye shadow, liner, and mascara can make eyes look sunken on TV. But defining the brows adds polish to the area without the negative side effects. Backstage at Miss Universe, makeup artists first clean up stray hairs above and below the arches, then fill and extend them. Rather than using a pencil, which can look severe and waxy, many pros prefer brow powder roughly the shade of the hair on the head. Using a small, stiff brush, they comb it into the brows using short strokes in the direction of hair growth.

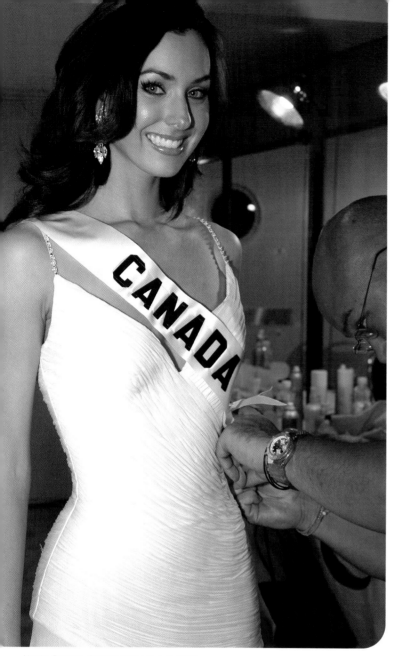

Natalie Glebova, Canada, Miss Universe 2005

# headlines

We'll admit it—until recently beauty queens were as notorious for their immovable hair as for their unflappable smiles. These days, pearly whites are still very much in fashion, but the helmet-like styles have all but disappeared. "Pageant women used to have this very crunchy Barbie thing going on," admits New York City hair guru John Barrett, the go-to guy for the reigning Miss Universe. "But in the last three or four years, they've definitely loosened up. Contestants tend to look like regular, ordinary, but very beautiful women. Most of them have sensual hair that actually moves."

## universal truth

Spotlights can make a few flyaways look like a fuzzy halo. Hairstylist Vernell Hooker and his colleagues backstage prefer Farouk's CHI ceramic curling irons, flat irons, and blow-dryers because they contain ions that seal cuticles. The result: Hair looks smoother and sleeker, even when the pressure—and the megawatt lighting—is on.

Natalie Glebova's lustrous locks didn't single-handedly score her the crown in Bangkok, but they sure didn't hurt. Farouk Systems hairstylist Vernell Hooker, who worked his magic on the raven-headed Canadian beauty, explains how he did it.

**Pump it up.** Every hairstyle falls a bit during the pageant, but Natalie's super-straight tresses were especially vulnerable. So Hooker started by building a sturdy foundation with a good spritzing of volumizer (in this case, Farouk Systems Infratexture) at the roots.

**Turn up the heat.** Hooker wrapped small sections around a hot curling iron, angling those pieces toward the hairline to create serious body and even more lift at the roots. He pinned each curl against the scalp until the hair cooled and set.

**Give it a hand.** After removing the pins, he broke up the curls by gently finger-combing. Because gravity took care of the longer pieces and ends of the hair, he used his hands to style waves in place around the face.

**Seal the deal.** To lock out humidity and lock in style, Hooker misted the entire head with Farouk's BioSilk finishing spray. A light-hold formula that still allows for movement, it contains silk particles for soft, natural-looking shine.

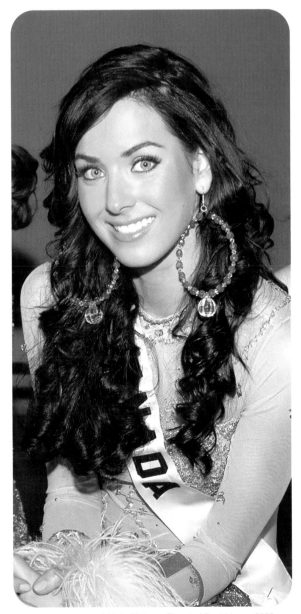

Natalie Glebova, Canada, Miss Universe 2005

# best tressed

Of course, the techniques that work magic on Natalie Glebova's thick, straight hair might spell doom for the fine-locked blonde in the neighboring chair. Here, broken down by hair type and texture, is a sampling of some of the ingenious tricks we noticed backstage.

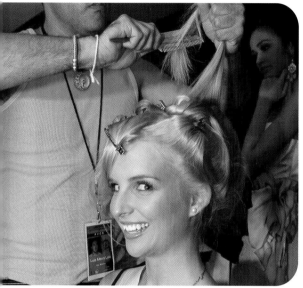

Michelle Guy, Australia, 2005 Miss Universe Contestant

## fine hair

### Look at the upside.
To make small hair bigger, blow-dry halfway, then flip the head over and finish the job while misting hair closest to the scalp with volumizing spray to lock in some root lift.

### Be a tease.
A little backcombing around the crown and nape of the neck adds fullness and body.

### Shine on.
Use shine spray containing silicone and silk to coat strands and keep frizz at bay.

### Be a smooth operator.
The best-kept secret: Bounce fabric softener sheets. Stylists drag them downward along the surface of the hair to smooth away fuzz just before showtime and between acts.

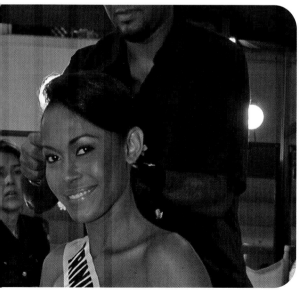

Magdalene Walcott, Trinidad & Tobago, 2005 Miss Universe Contestant

## african hair

### Pump some iron.
For locks that haven't been chemically relaxed, flat irons do double duty: The pros twist the iron as they drag it through small sections of hair. This smoothes the kinks while simultaneously creating large waves.

### Extend yourself.
Extensions and weaves were *huge* in Bangkok. Stylists added straight and curled pieces (to match the girl's own hair texture) at the crown of the head and above the nape to add fullness and flowing length.

### Add loads of luster.
African hair tends to be on the dry side. A final shot of shine spray just before showtime restores sheen, making tresses look soft, hydrated, and healthy.

## asian hair

**Style in seconds—flat.** Because of their coarse texture, unruly pieces are especially obvious. The stylists' secrets to keeping them in check: Moisten fingertips with a pomade such as Farouk Twisted Fiber, pinch the misbehaving strands together with the rest of the hair until the whole section is lying flat, and press with a flat iron.

**Turn up the gloss.** An allover misting with shine spray enhances the natural gloss Asian hair is famous for.

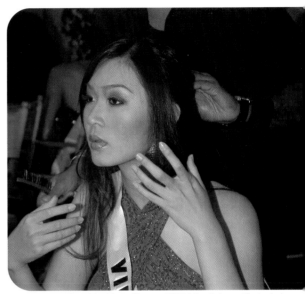

Pham Thu Hang, Vietnam, 2005 Miss Universe Contestant

## full hair

**Work backward.** Latina women are often blessed with loads of gorgeous hair. The challenge is to keep it from overwhelming an equally gorgeous face. A few Velcro rollers popped along the hairline for ten minutes direct those tresses backward—without sacrificing the volume.

**Go halfway.** Pinning up only the front half of the hair at the crown shows off the face while preserving the mane's natural body in back.

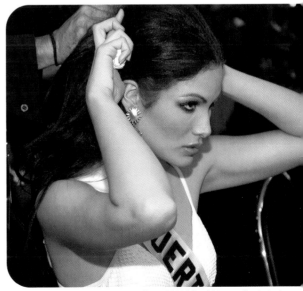

Cynthia Olavarria, Puerto Rico, 2005 Miss Universe Contestant

PART 2

# everyday beauty

# the body beautiful

## Martha Vasconcellos, Brazil, Miss Universe 1968

Martha Vasconcellos was a perfect angel as a teenager in Bahia, Brazil, during the late sixties. No broken curfews. No sneaking cigarettes in the bathroom. "I was very obedient," she says. "There was never any adolescent craziness. I didn't give my parents any trouble." Then she discovered beauty pageants.

When Martha was first invited to a local competition, at age fourteen, her father put his foot down. "He was a lawyer for the government and very well known in Brazil," she recalls. "He said 'No!' For him, this was too much exposure and it was out of the family plans." She obeyed him, at first, until the pageant bug became too much for her to withstand. Against her father's wishes, she entered a small pageant in town—and won. Just for kicks, she strutted her stuff in Rio de Janeiro—and stole that crown, too. "Then came Miss Brazil," Martha says. "When I won it, I was very surprised. My father wanted to kill me. These pageants were my form of rebellion."

She rebelled all the way to Miami, the site of the 1968 Miss Universe competition—and soon garnered enough attention from pageant officials to distract her from the drama back home. "When they measured me for my swimsuit size, they asked me to take off my bra—I think they thought I was stuffing it with something!" she says. Her curvy figure, of course, was 100 percent Martha, and she easily walked away with the crown.

This Latina beauty married her childhood sweetheart in Bahia and raised her family there, also working for many years in the business world. But after becoming deeply interested in psychoanalysis, she eventually left Brazil to start a new career on her own in the USA as a psychotherapist.

Nearly forty years later, the former Miss Universe's body is still among her greatest assets. She's meticulous about keeping every square inch moisturized and protected from the sun. As for those famous curves: "I take very good care of them," says Martha. "When I wake up, the first thing I do is put on a bra. And when I was pregnant, I never slept without one. I am a woman—I won't be happy if my body looks like hell."

Here's your ticket to loving the skin you're in.

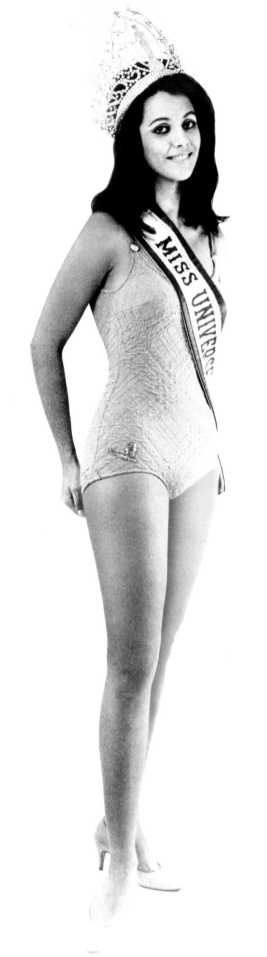

# you big softie

A lot has changed since Martha Vasconcellos's beauty queen days, but her body remains just as supple. Because cold weather, harsh cleansing, and age can take a toll on the skin's protective lipid barrier (leading to flakes and redness), Martha shores it up with a generous dollop of moisturizer the minute she steps out of the shower. Here, more secrets to beautifying your bod.

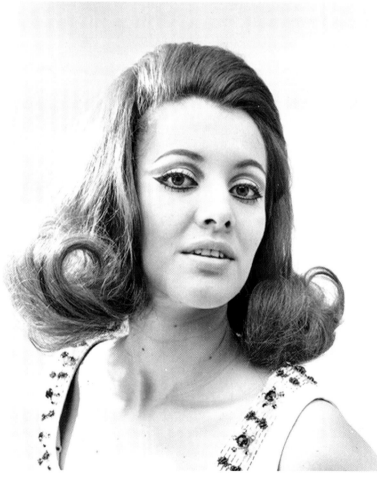

Martha Vasconcellos, Brazil, Miss Universe 1968

Shower smart. Soaking too long in soap lather and hot water can literally wash your skin's natural oils down the drain, which is why experts advise limiting shower time to no more than fifteen minutes and keeping the water as tepid as possible. Because bar soaps tend to be more drying than creamy, liquid varieties, Martha coddles her skin with organic Jason Satin Soap with aloe vera, which she picks up at her local yoga studio. "The label says it's for the hands and face," she says. "So I figure it must be very mild and gentle."

Use the right goop. Slather moisturizer over damp skin, within minutes of showering. The formula should contain plenty of occlusive ingredients, such as petrolatum and shea butter, to seal that shower water into the skin. But make sure it's also rich in humectants, such as glycerin, hyaluronic acid, and urea, which draw in more water molecules. Severely dry areas, such as the knees, elbows, and hands, usually deserve more concentrated formulas. The trick to finding a suitable moisturizer for these areas is to turn the closed bottle upside down and watch how it falls to the bottom. The slower it falls, the richer the formula. And in general, ointments are richer than creams, which are richer than lotions.

Scrub a dub. The flakes and dead skin cells that build up, especially during the winter months, are not only unsightly—but also prevent moisturizer from absorbing properly. And that can lead to more flakes. End the vicious cycle by gently exfoliating with a grainy scrub once every week or two, or use a moisturizer containing alpha hydroxy acids every few days. The exception: Very red or scaly skin can't handle harsh cleansers, so stick to creamy body washes and AHA-free moisturizers until the dry patches heal.

Baby your bod. When skin is so dry it hurts, see a dermatologist, who can prescribe a medicated heavy-duty moisturizer. Martha's personal prescription for rough, cracked feet: diaper rash cream. "It's called A+D Original Ointment and it's about $10 for a big pot," she says. "Before cleaning the house, I rub the ointment all over my feet, then put on thick socks. By the time I'm done, my skin is so soft, you just can't imagine!"

Take your medicine. Drinking eight glasses of water daily certainly can't hurt your skin, but swallowing the right supplements with your water can certainly help it. Some experts believe that capsules containing lecithin (also found in spinach, eggs, and soy) and essential fatty acids such as fish oil, flaxseed oil, and evening primrose oil help replenish the skin's lipid barrier.

Sleep yourself smooth. Moisture loss doesn't stop when you hit the hay, which is why it's wise to coat yourself in body cream before turning in for the night. Keeping a humidifier in the bedroom will also help keep skin hydrated.

# light savers

Growing up in Brazil, Martha Vasconcellos spent half the year baking to a golden brown. "I'd go home for lunch when the sun was strongest, put on my bikini, and lay out by the swimming pool," she recalls. Now, of course, Martha is wiser—and quite a bit paler. She knows that the sun's ultraviolet rays can cause skin cancer, not to mention wrinkles, blotches, and other signs of aging. "Ten years ago," she says, "I stopped sunning. I buy an SPF 45—the kind designed for babies—because it's gentle. When I go back to the beaches of Brazil, I reapply it every time I get out of the water. Now I'm white as snow."

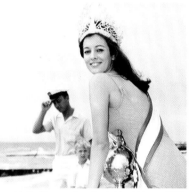

Martha Vasconcellos, Brazil, Miss Universe 1968

**The Lingo:**
The SPF number

**Translation:** This measures how well the lotion shields against UVB—the rays that cause sunburns and skin cancer. Properly applied, an SPF 15 blocks 94 percent of those rays for about two hours. Higher numbers shield you for longer—though the products also tend to be thicker and stickier. One word of caution: SPF does not refer to how well the formula protects against UVA light, the rays responsible for wrinkles and that also contribute to cancer. So far, the FDA hasn't approved a universal way to measure this.

**The Lingo:**
Broad-spectrum

**Translation:** This is your cue that the formula guards against both UVA and UVB rays, probably with ingredients such as zinc oxide, avobenzone (the trademarked name is Parsol 1789), and titanium dioxide.

**The Lingo:**
Physical sunblock

**Translation:** The two most effective are zinc oxide and titanium dioxide. Ground into tiny particles, these sit on top of the skin and reflect light away. While physical blockers tend to feel chalky and thick, some newer formulas contain microfine particles that glide on smoothly without leaving a white residue.

**The Lingo:**
Chemical sunblock

**Translation:** The best one right now is avobenzone (Parsol 1789), which interacts with skin cells to absorb UV rays. Most experts advise choosing a sunscreen with a combination of chemical and physical blockers—unless you have very sensitive skin, which can be irritated by chemical ingredients.

# operation application

Porntip "Bui" Nakhirunkanok Simon (Thailand, Miss Universe 1988) says that in her native Thailand any hint of sun exposure is frowned upon. "Sun spots are seen as a sign that you've been working out in the fields," she says. "The Thai language doesn't even have a word for *tan.*" The secret to her radiant, blotch-free bod is about more than just applying sunscreen—it's about knowing how to rub it in right. Here are some tricks for protecting your skin with sunscreen.

**Think ahead.** Rub sunscreen into the skin twenty minutes before going outside, so the active ingredients have time to work.

**Lay it on thick.** It takes a teaspoon of sunscreen to properly protect the face, and the equivalent of a shot glass for the entire body, including the face. If your SPF 45 feels too gloppy or chalky, switch to a lower number. Better to wear a thick coat of an SPF 15 than a wimpy layer of the strong stuff.

**Then do it again.** Sunscreen breaks down with exposure to sweat, water, and even sunlight. So reapply every two hours you're outside—and immediately after swimming.

**Use it, then lose it.** You may need reading glasses to decode the expiration date, but it's worth it. Sunscreen can start to lose effectiveness after several months, so it's a good idea to replace your stash every season. Besides, experts say that if you're still dipping into the same tube at the end of the summer that you bought at the beginning, you're not using enough.

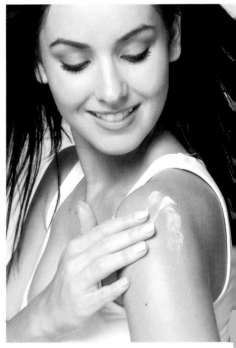

Natalie Glebova, Canada, Miss Universe 2005

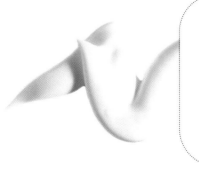

## universal truth

Damaging ultraviolet rays have no trouble traveling through car and airplane windows. To keep her hands looking young and blotch-free, Bui Simon puts on plenty of Clarins Age Control Hand Lotion SPF 15 before gripping the steering wheel. And to protect her face, neck, and arms while flying the friendly skies, she notes, "that's what those window shades are for."

# the faux glow

Miss Universe hopefuls know there's no such thing as a safe tan—but they also know that even the most gorgeous skin can look pasty and washed out under stage lights. What's a beauty queen to do? "Self-tanner, all over the body, is an almost compulsory part of the pageant," says CoverGirl makeup artist B.J. Gillian, who works backstage during the competition. "Ninety-nine percent of the time, that wonderfully rich skin you see on television is a result of artificial technology." For some women, that means visiting a Mystic Tan booth (thousands of salons feature them), which airbrushes the body with a flawless, UV-free film of self-tanner that lasts about a week. For those who prefer to apply it themselves, straight from the tube, Gillian recommends the following technique.

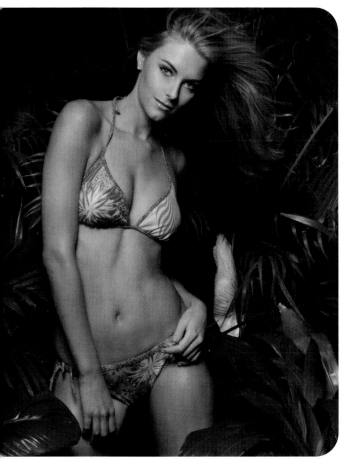

Jennifer Hawkins, Australia, Miss Universe 2004

Start in the shower. Self-tanner works by dying the surface layers of the skin. If your body is flaky or thicker in some areas, that dye will cling unevenly, and "you'll look like you were rolling around in iron oxide," says Gillian, who recommends first running a wet washcloth or soft loofah over the entire body in the shower. "Focus your scrubbing on the roughest areas, like the knees, heels, and knuckles. And use a moisturizing cleanser to keep skin supple and prevent flakes." When you step out of the shower, gently blot the body dry with a fluffy towel. Self-tanner is best applied when skin is ever so slightly moist.

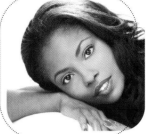
**Use a light hand.** Whether or not you're competing for a crown, self-tanner is best applied sparingly, as the formula's true shade can take hours to fully develop. "Think of it as a rare, precious cream," says Gillian. "It should disappear quickly into your skin. If it takes more than four to five minutes to dry, you've probably put on too much. You can always put on another layer if you decide you're not bronze enough—but if you overdo it on the first application, you'll have to wait days for it to fade."

**Do the rough stuff last.** Rub a thin, even coat of self-tanner over the arms, legs, and torso—saving thick-skinned spots, such as elbows, knees, and heels, for the end. "These areas will grab the color most easily, so by the time you get to them, you should have almost no self-tanner on your hands at all," says Gillian. "And you're best off enlisting a partner to do the tough-to-reach areas like your back. Most of the Miss Universe girls have their moms or roommates do it."

**Wash up.** The palms are one of the roughest parts of the body, so it's especially important that you thoroughly wash your hands the minute you put down the self-tanner tube. Otherwise, you'll spend the next five days looking as if you played in mud. Not a good look.

**Take care of the color.** The best way to maximize a self-tanner's staying power: Lay off the exfoliating scrubs and be sure to moisturize. "If you let skin dry out, the color will begin to wear off unevenly," cautions Gillian. Apply a hydrating cream in the morning and at bedtime.

**Don't ditch the SPF.** A fake bake, unlike the real thing, will not protect you from the sun's harmful rays. "Even if you look like a bronze goddess, you should apply sunscreen like you're the palest girl on the beach," says Gillian.

# hair today, gone tomorrow

Martha Vasconcellos used to wax her bikini area religiously—until she grew fed up with the ingrown hairs. And, let's face it, plenty of us can relate. Those pimple-like bumps that form when hair curls back under the surface of the skin are especially common after waxing spots where the hair is coarse. These days, Martha's bikini-line is beautifully bare, thanks to several rounds of electrolysis, a treatment in which an aesthetician destroys individual hair follicles with electric current delivered through a fine needle. While results are permanent after several sessions, it's tedious work—which is why more and more women are opting for laser hair removal instead.

New York City dermatologist Cheryl Thellman-Karcher, who keeps reigning Miss Universes glowing from head to toe, notes many of today's contestants enter as fans of the razor, hot wax, or depilatory—but "most of them end up switching to the laser," she says. "You're dealing with all different types of skin in this pageant, and the newest lasers can treat any of them. That said, even the most high-tech treatments have their drawbacks—most significantly, the cost involved. Thellman-Karcher guides us through the most popular fuzz busters.

## shaving

How it works: For the closest shave, choose a manual (nonelectric) razor with a new blade. Thellman-Karcher tells patients to soak in a warm tub first, then "lather with a very creamy shaving cream" to minimize irritation. Using a razor with a pivoted, springy head and at least two blades will also help ensure the best shave.

Consider it for: Legs and underarms. Shaving is an extremely efficient way to eliminate large swaths of hair growth. These areas are also less prone to ingrowns, which shaving can induce.

Expect to pay: About $7.50 for a pack of ten disposable Gillette Daisy Ultragrip razors. A Gillette Venus Divine nondisposable razor is about $10.

Results: Smooth skin within minutes—and stubbly regrowth within a day or two.

The pleasure: It's cheap, simple, and speedy.

The pain: Aside from the occasional nick, very little—unless you're prone to the unsightly red bumps commonly known as razor burn, which can be caused by irritation from shaving. For those women, Thellman-Karcher generally recommends intermittent treatment with a mild steroid cream. Talk to your doctor about the best product and course of treatment for you. Foliculitis, an infection that sometimes crops up after shaving, can be soothed with a prescription antibiotic lotion.

## depilatory

How it works: These creams, mousses, and lotions contain chemicals that dissolve hair just below the skin's surface.

Consider it for: Anywhere, as long as it's not near the eyes, mouth, or other mucous membranes. But if you have sensitive skin, you might want to keep it away from your upper lip and other facial areas. A red, blotchy mustache isn't any better than a fuzzy one!

Expect to pay: Nair 4-Minute Lotion Cucumber Melon Hair Remover is about $4.50.

Results: Most do a decent job of whisking away hair, but results can be patchy. And the fuzz typically returns nearly as quickly as it does after shaving.

The pleasure: Smooth legs in minutes, without razor burn.

The pain: Some formulas have a pretty heinous chemical stench—which is why some versions try to mask it with scents of cucumber and melon. The actual pain is usually zilch, unless you happen to have sensitive skin, in which case you may feel some stinging.

## waxing

**How it works:** No mincing words here: Whether done in the salon or at home, wax (usually attached to a strip of cloth) yanks hair out by the roots.

**Consider it for:** Anywhere—but keep in mind hair has to be at least a quarter inch long. Doing a small area such as the upper lip obviously has a lower ouch factor, but Thellman-Karcher offers this caveat: "The skin there is so thin and gentle that waxing can irritate it and sometimes cause post-inflammatory hyperpigmentation. Some girls end up with a brown mustache!" Bleaching creams usually clear up the splotches, but those who do wax the area would be wise to use a steroid cream immediately after treatment—ask your doctor to prescribe one—then stay out of the sun for about a week. If you're taking topical retinoids or Accutane, consult your dermatologist before waxing.

**Expect to pay:** Legs can run up to $100, while the upper lip can be less than $10. That's assuming you do it in a salon (not in your bathroom), which most experts recommend.

**Results:** Because hair is removed at the root, skin can stay bare for up to six weeks.

**The pleasure:** Waxing injures the root, so regrowth is often finer. That means prickly stubble is less of a problem. The process is also fairly quick and long lasting, and it won't tax your pocketbook too much.

**The pain:** Aside from the undeniable discomfort when the wax is ripped off, many women experience painful ingrown hairs during the weeks after. To ease the former, pop an aspirin or apply a prescription numbing cream before going to the salon. Then use a clean, wet washcloth to gently exfoliate waxed areas daily to release trapped hairs and prevent ingrowns.

## electrolysis

**How it works:** An aesthetician's needle pumps electrical current into each hair follicle one by one, destroying them.

**Consider it for:** Small areas, such as the upper lip and brow.

**Expect to pay:** About $25 to $50 per fifteen-minute session.

**Results:** Permanent hair removal requires several months of treatment, as hair grows in different cycles and some follicles may be dormant during any one electrolysis session.

**The pleasure:** "Eventually you get permanent hair removal," says Thellman-Karcher. "And that's hard to find."

**The pain:** The needle insertion—over and over again—can sting and cause mild irritation. Topical numbing cream or a preemptive aspirin can help. And again, because only one follicle is treated at a time, the process can be painfully slow.

## lasers and other light sources

**How it works:** Lasers (such as the Lyra and Alexandrite) and a related treatment called Intense Pulsed Light deliver energy that heats and destroys hair follicles.

**Consider it for:** Those with fair skin and dark hair respond best, but the latest devices also work (albeit not as well) on dark skin and very light hair. Anyone using topical retinoids or Accutane should consult her dermatologist before considering treatment.

**Expect to pay:** Several hundred to several thousand dollars per treatment.

**Results:** Most women need four to eight sessions, two to three weeks apart, to see permanent reduction in fuzz.

**The pleasure:** Often, hair is mostly gone for good after several months of treatment. And if you do experience regrowth, the hair will be sparser and less coarse.

**The pain:** Mild discomfort—and a fairly major drain on your wallet.

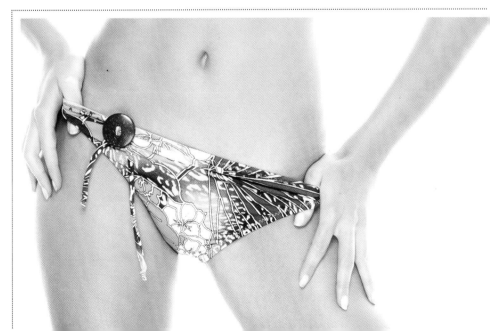

# the sleek physique

During the three weeks leading up to the 2005 Miss Universe competition, the eighty-one contestants were ping-ponging to so many events, parties, and photo shoots that they barely had time to brush their teeth, let alone sneak in a workout. But somehow Natalie Glebova (Canada, Miss Universe 2005) managed to turn her hotel room into a makeshift gym. "I had a really wonderful personal trainer before I left for Thailand, and he gave me some exercises and three-pound weights that I could take anywhere," she says. Hundreds of sit-ups and leg raises later, Natalie was standing in a white bikini before a worldwide audience of almost one billion. And she felt proud.

Kudos to Natalie. Experts confirm that the best fitness formula is one that fits within *your* lifestyle. They advise against making unrealistic demands on your body, and encourage keeping your workouts portable and interesting so that you don't tire of them easily. Because let's face it—it doesn't matter how intense your workouts are if you don't keep them up.

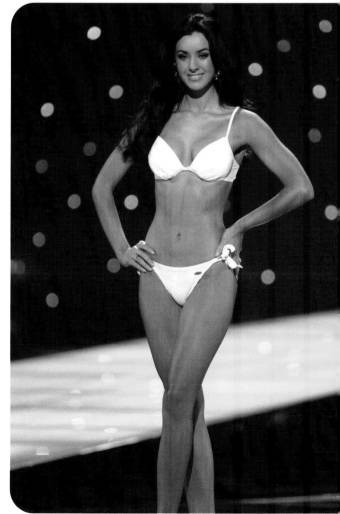

Natalie Glebova, Canada, Miss Universe 2005

# shape-up strategies

Clayton James and Robert "Sid" Sidbury, trainers at the Reebok Sports Club in New York City, are charged with keeping reigning Miss Universes beautifully buff. And while it seems like a big job, they say getting on the fast track to fit boils down to six simple secrets.

**Make it a vacation.** If you view exercise as a chore, it will become a chore. Sidbury says that most of his crown-wearing clients are so insanely busy that "training is like a getaway for them—a way to unwind between all of their appearances." What better way to shake off the daily grind than to crank up the iPod and embrace your sweaty side?

**Get creative.** It's easy to feel intimidated by the wealth of workout contraptions out there (stability ball, anyone?). But force yourself to sample as many as possible. "If you're always running," says Sidbury, "give your joints a rest and hop on your bike or take out a jump rope." Not only will you keep boredom at bay, but you'll challenge your body in new ways—a surefire cure for those pesky weight-loss plateaus.

**Get high—then low.** When James put Jennifer Hawkins (Australia, Miss Universe 2005) on the treadmill, he had her do a combination of walking and jogging. The advantage to this kind of interval training: Downshifting the pace every few minutes staves off exhaustion so you keep going for longer than you would if you were jogging the whole time. And that can mean only good things for your metabolism.

**Don't do one without the other.** We're talking cardio and strength training here. Exercises that leave you winded (jogging, power walking, stairclimbing, cycling) are essential for good heart health and for instant calorie burn. But don't forget strength training (yoga, Pilates, dumbbells, and other weights), which tones and firms your arms, legs, abs, and back. And the more lean muscle mass you have, the higher your resting metabolism (the number of calories you burn when you're vegging in front of the TV).

**Know it's not all or nothing.** Too tired to do your full workout? Instead of ditching the gym entirely, aim at completing half your routine. A little movement is better than none. And besides, once you get into the exercise groove, you may not be able to quit!

**Take it with you.** To make sure their pageant-winning clients don't lose momentum while they're traveling (which is pretty much all the time), James and Sidbury teach them how to use exercise bands, jump ropes, and even hotel furniture as a makeshift gym. Then again, most hotels have pretty spiffy workout rooms of their own—and they're usually blessedly empty.

# you're at the gym—now what?

James adds one more component to the cardio and strength training equation: stretching. To him, a perfect workout session entails twenty to twenty-five minutes on the elliptical trainer, treadmill, or bike; twenty minutes of squats, weights, Pilates, and other muscle-building moves; and twenty minutes of good stretching. To reap the rewards of interval training, try blasting through the cardio portion in intense three-to-four-minute bursts, with stretching and strength training in between. Shoot for three to four workouts per week. While Natalie Glebova is usually far too busy to fit in daily routines, she incorporates cardio, strength training, and stretching into her workouts whenever possible.

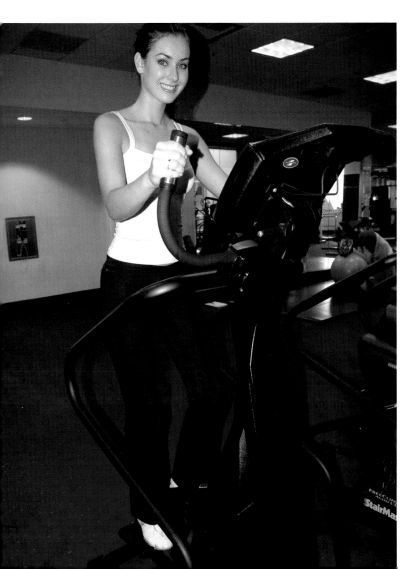

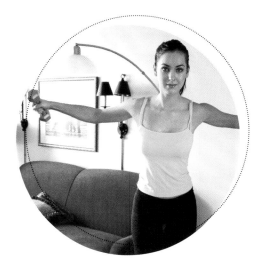

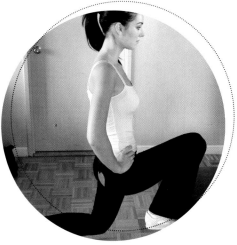

Natalie Gleb
Canada, Miss Universe 2

## in her own words

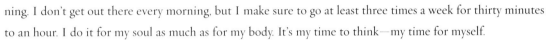

Yvonne Agneta-Ryding
Sweden, Miss Universe 1984

"Today, women my age have to deal with family, working life, and the stress of fitting in workouts on top of that. I like to make exercise as enjoyable as possible—if you're stressed about running on those machines every day, what's the point? I get a lot of positive energy from being outside in the woods, so that's where I do a lot of my exercising. It could be power walking, it could be running. I don't get out there every morning, but I make sure to go at least three times a week for thirty minutes to an hour. I do it for my soul as much as for my body. It's my time to think—my time for myself.

"As for food, I think women know what we should and shouldn't eat. But I have two very young girls, and I always try to express how important it is to actually have breakfast, lunch, and dinner. You can't just live on vitamin pills. I'm forty-two, and I really believe in enjoying life. On weekends, I eat dessert and try to keep the rest of my meals as nutritious—and tasty—as possible."

—Yvonne Agneta-Ryding, Sweden, Miss Universe 1984

## one day at yvonne's table

Breakfast: Low-fat yogurt with whole-grain, high-fiber bread and coffee.

Mid-morning snack: Piece of fruit.

Lunch: Large salad with serving of chicken or fish. ("I skip the potatoes and pasta because they make me tired," she says.)

Mid-afternoon snack: Coffee, a piece of fruit with crackers, and an occasional small hunk of chocolate.

Dinner: Roast chicken or salmon with a salad on the side.

Dessert: White chocolate mousse with wild strawberry sauce.

# the moves

There are countless ways to strengthen and tone your body. Some use your own weight as resistance, while others employ dumbbells or heavy gym equipment. Below, Robert Sidbury walks us through a few of the moves he uses to keep Natalie Glebova looking lean and lovely. Note that, for exercises involving dumbbells, Natalie usually uses three-to-five pound weights. You should use weights that feel challenging after twelve repetitions.

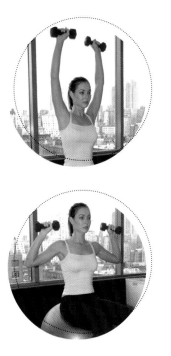

**Dumbbell shoulder press:** Works the anterior and middle deltoids. If you use a stability ball, you'll also work your core muscles—abdominals and middle and lower back.

1. Sit upright on a stability ball (or chair, if no ball is available) with your feet shoulder-width apart.

2. Get into starting position by raising the dumbbells to shoulder height, with elbows out and palms facing out.

3. Press your arms over your head so that they are straight.

4. Bring your arms back down to starting position.

5. Lift your arms again. Continue for three sets of twelve. Alternate each set with a set of bicep curls (see next page).

## universal truth

Sidbury makes sure to balance these simple upper-body moves with exercises that work the lower body. He usually starts Natalie off by having her walk briskly on the treadmill for eight minutes at a steep incline. While this is primarily geared toward keeping her heart rate up and burning calories, it tones the legs as well. Sidbury also has Natalie do squats and lunges while holding five-pound weights, as well as side leg raises.

Bicep curl: Works the biceps. If you use a stability ball, you also work the core muscles.

1. Sitting upright on a stability ball with your back straight and head up, hold a dumbbell in each hand.

2. Let your arms hang at your sides.

3. Keeping your elbows close to the body, curl your arms up so that the weights almost touch your shoulders.

4. Slowly lower your arms and return them to your sides. Repeat for three sets of twelve. Alternate each set with a set of dumbbell shoulder presses (left).

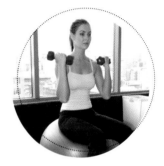

Side raise: Works the middle deltoid muscle group.

1. Holding a dumbbell in each hand, let your arms hang at your sides.

2. Keep your arms straight with a slight bend in the elbows as you raise them until they're level with your shoulders.

3. Lower your arms back to your sides. Repeat for three sets of twelve.

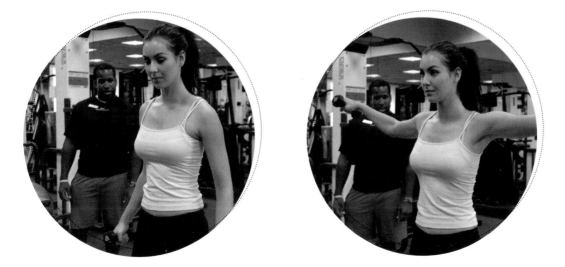

# flawless skin

## Jennifer Hawkins, Australia, Miss Universe 2004

Aussie women have a knack for looking beautiful without even trying—whether they're striding into a cocktail party or sweating on a treadmill. And Jennifer Hawkins is certainly no exception. Growing up, she was just as comfortable surfing waves on a long board as modeling in front of cameras, approaching each venture with effortless grace and polish. "I turned up at model castings in jeans, flip-flops, and no makeup," she recalls. "That's how I liked it."

Jennifer was able to maintain her low-key style when she entered (and won) the Miss Australia pageant at age twenty. But when she flew off to Ecuador to compete for Miss Universe (her first trip away from her home continent), it was a whole new ball game. During the three weeks of preliminary competitions leading up to the big contest, she swapped her sandals for stilettos and learned to love (or at least tolerate) the feel of lipstick and heavy foundation on her face. "I was wearing evening gowns all the time over there," says Jennifer. "In Australia, you don't wear a long dress unless you're a bridesmaid." But even with the makeup and gowns, Jennifer refused to worry much about wooing her audience. "I took my mom's advice," she says. "Just be yourself and have fun." Clearly, it worked.

Jennifer continues to heed her mother's wise words. Since turning in her crown last year, she's reunited with her surfboard and eased up on the makeup, allowing her freshly scrubbed Aussie glow to show more than ever. But looking naturally flawless means Jennifer can't be quite so laid back about one area: skincare. She doesn't apply many products to her face but makes sure those she does use won't clog her pores. "I have to use moisturizer that's oil-free," she once told *Shop Til You Drop* magazine. "Otherwise my skin will break out. The brand isn't important to me, it just can't have any oil." And she'd never *think* of hitting the hay before washing her face and putting on eye cream. In other words, it takes a bit of work to attain—and maintain—a seemingly effortlessly beautiful complexion.

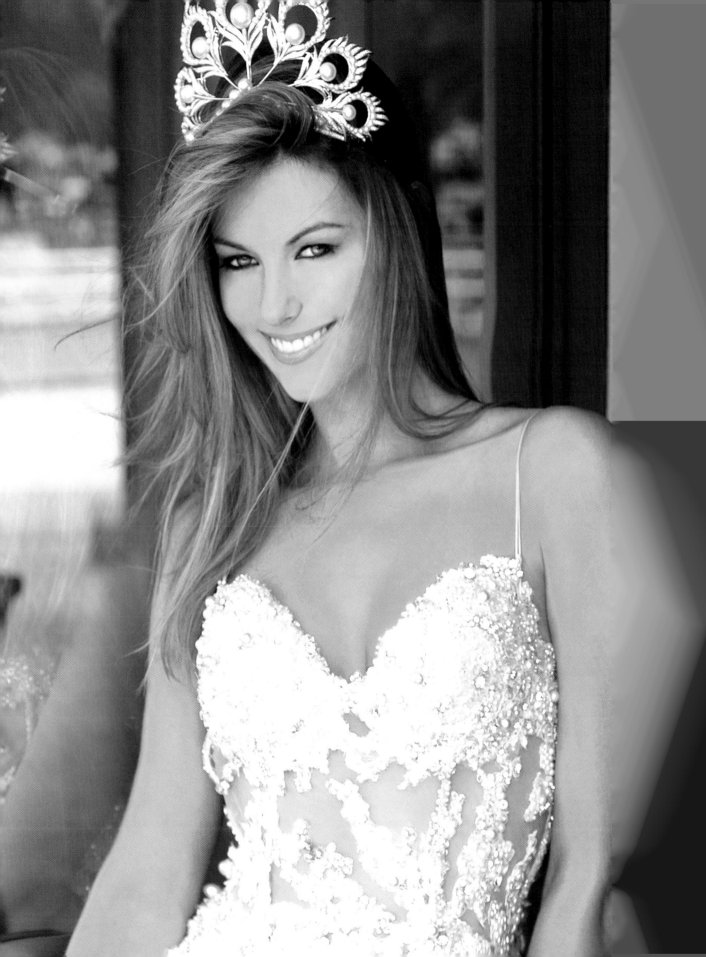

# the doctor is in

Anyone who thinks Miss Universe doesn't have skin problems should talk to New York City dermatologist Cheryl Thellman-Karcher, the woman who helps the world's crowned beauties put their best face forward. Tending to all types of complexions—from Irish to Latina, oily to flaky—she says that even titleholders who grew up with problem-free skin usually encounter some sort of facial issue during their reign. And is it any wonder? For one action-packed year, these women are living under hot spotlights, caking on makeup, logging thousands of frequent-flyer miles, and getting far less sleep than they should. "The number one problem I see is acne," says the dermatologist, who also treats her fair share of facial blotches, brown spots, and even fine lines.

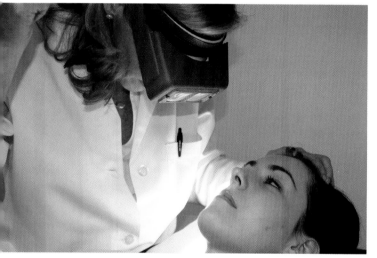

Dermatologist Cheryl Thellman-Karcher
with Natalie Glebova, Canada, Miss Universe 2005

When she examines an entering Miss Universe for the first time, Thellman-Karcher asks her to bring her supply of skin products along—and suggests that all women do the same when they visit a dermatologist. "That way, I can analyze exactly what they're using," she says. "Often, their at-home regimen is part of the problem." This is a good rule of thumb for anyone—pageant-bound or not. And even if you don't go to a dermatologist, it's a good idea to assess your own skin type to make sure your products are doing everything they can for your complexion.

## what's your type?

It's best to have a dermatologist analyze your skin for any hidden issues, but you can do a pretty good job assessing your own complexion by examining it after cleansing with a mild soap or wash. Wait an hour or so after rinsing, then ask yourself:

*Do I feel greasy?* If you already have the urge to lather up again—especially around your forehead and nose—you probably have oily skin. Large pores are another dead giveaway.

*Do I feel tight?* If your face feels taut, looks papery, or is flaking in spots, your complexion is dry.

*Do I feel unsure?* If your cheeks feel a little dry and your T-zone (forehead, nose, and chin) is shiny, you, like most women, have combination skin.

*Do I feel itchy or tingly?* If your face is blotchy, red, or hurts slightly, you probably have sensitive skin.

*Do I feel fine?* If your skin still looks velvety and untroubled, you have normal skin. Truly one of the lucky ones!

*Do I feel mature?* As you move into your thirties and beyond, skin tends to lose fat, collagen, and elasticity. This leads to more fine lines and a papery, crepe-like texture. Mature skin is usually dry.

Asked about her favorite beauty routine, Deborah Carthy-Deu (Puerto Rico, Miss Universe 1985) doesn't miss a beat. "Living in the tropics, I feel great every time I'm able to clean my skin," she says. Women living around the globe can surely relate. Regularly washing the face is the best preemptive strike against a host of complexion problems. Lather up at bedtime to completely remove makeup, excess surface oil, and pollutants that have settled on the skin throughout the day. Cleansing again in the morning whisks away any oil that your pores have pumped out overnight—not to mention the grime your cheeks have picked up from pressing against your pillow for seven hours. (If you have very dry skin, you might consider rinsing without cleanser in the AM.) Here, a basic guide to washing up.

**Splish, splash.** Moisten the face with at least ten splashes of lukewarm water. Extremely hot or cold water can dry or irritate the skin. If you have dry skin, you may want to use a creamy cleanser that wipes on and off without water.

**Come clean.** Using small circular motions, massage cleanser into the face. Pay special attention to the T-zone—especially the area around the nose—where oil and grime tend to accumulate. Thellman-Karcher tells most patients to use a mild, gentle cleanser because anything too harsh can strip away the skin's natural lipid barrier, leaving it open to irritation. Those with very oily or acne-prone skin should look for a formula that doesn't leave a moisturizing film behind—and might try a cleanser containing salicylic acid, provided it doesn't leave the skin dry or blotchy. Sensitive types do best with a cleanser containing polyethylene glycol, which does not penetrate the skin. And women with very dry skin should look for a nonfoaming creamy cleanser with moisturizers that replenish the skin's lipid barrier.

**Rinse.** Splash again with lukewarm water, at least twelve to fifteen times or until no residue is left on the skin. Pat face dry with a clean cloth or towel.

**Earn extra credit.** Wait at least five minutes (but fifteen minutes is better) for your skin to dry thoroughly. Exactly what you apply at this point depends on time of day and type of skin. In the morning, sunscreen is a must—an oil-free gel for oily skin, a lotion for normal skin, a moisturizing cream with sunscreen for dry skin. Bedtime is the ideal hour for treatment products, such as topical vitamins, alpha hydroxy acids (AHAs), and retinoids, because sunlight can render many of these ingredients ineffective. Some treatment ingredients, such as AHAs, can make the skin more sensitive to sunlight. So whether your cream is designed to fight fine lines or reduce ultraviolet light damage, your face will benefit most if you put it on at night.

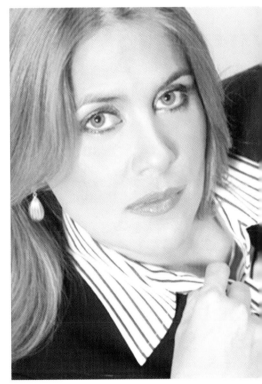

Deborah Carthy-Deu, Puerto Rico, Miss Universe 1985

# complexion quandary number 1: acne

Acne is enemy number one among Thellman-Karcher's pageant-winning patients—but it can strike any woman at any point in her life. Thankfully, the arsenal of pimple-fighting weapons is stronger and more effective than ever. The first step to keeping blemishes at bay is to understand why they appear in the first place. Step two is finding the right treatment as early as possible to minimize the chance of scarring—both physical and emotional.

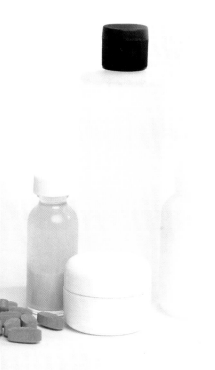

## why acne happens

Let's get one thing straight—there's no proof that eating chocolate or fried foods causes a breakout. (Although if you notice that a particular food seems to make you break out, see if it makes a difference to cut it from your diet for a month.) Here's what doctors know *does* cause acne.

**Excess oil production.** While stress and genetics can affect the skin's oil (or sebum) levels, they're typically triggered by hormonal changes. That's why acne is common not only during adolescence, but also throughout the thirties and forties, when pregnancy, birth control pills, and menopause are wreaking havoc with hormone levels.

**Dead skin cells.** Starting in puberty, the inside of an oil (or sebaceous) gland start to shed dead skin more rapidly. When those skin cells mix with an increased amount of sebum, that thick, sticky mixture can form a plug—which becomes a blackhead or a whitehead.

**Bacteria.** To further complicate matters, bacteria normally present in the skin, called *p. acnes,* tend to multiply inside clogged sebaceous glands, producing substances that irritate the surrounding area. The gland continues to swell, and may burst, spreading the inflammation to surrounding skin. This is what causes cystic acne—the type most likely to leave long-term pigmentation and permanent pockmark scars behind.

**universal truth** ♛ Last-minute flights around the globe, daily workouts with personal trainers, appearances at the United Nations—while it may be glamorous being Miss Universe, it's also super-stressful. Stress can increase hormonal activity, leading to higher levels of hormones called androgens, the big culprits behind pimples, according to Thellman-Karcher. She advises acne-prone patients to try stress-reducing activities such as yoga as an adjunct to any zit-fighting medications they're using.

**is it really acne?** One more reason to consult an expert before self-treating your pimples: They may not be pimples at all. Rosacea is a condition that often mimics acne. In the early stages, patients flush easily around their nose and cheeks—then tend to develop pimple-like bumps in those areas. Dermatologists believe rosacea is caused primarily by bacteria. It's made worse by stress, and unlike acne, it's definitely exacerbated by certain foods such as chocolate, red wine, hot drinks, and anything very spicy. Most cases respond to a topical treatment called Metrogel. And several rounds of laser therapy can zap away the facial flushes (actually caused by broken blood vessels), which can become permanent in the condition's late stages.

# plan of attack

An acne breakout can spell disaster for a pageant contestant. For the rest of us, it can put a serious damper on a hot date, a job interview, or even an ordinary trip to the grocery store. Fortunately, the myriad of treatments available now means that if one doesn't work, there's always another cream, pill, or therapy to try. The best rule of thumb when battling blemishes, says Thellman-Karcher, is to start with the gentler, less invasive options and work up from there. And because most of these treatments can take weeks or even months to work, remember to be patient.

The drugstore darlings. For the occasional zit, over-the-counter products containing benzoyl peroxide (a drying agent that kills bacteria) or salicylic acid (a beta hydroxy acid that dissolves pore-clogging dead skin cells) may do the trick. As long as it doesn't irritate your skin, swab a gentle, alcohol-free toner with salicylic acid over your entire face after cleansing before bed. Then spot-treat acne-prone areas with a benzoyl peroxide cream. Be sure any products you're using on the skin are oil-free and labeled *noncomedogenic* (meaning "non-pore-clogging").

The tougher topicals. If over-the-counter treatments don't work, your dermatologist might prescribe a cream or lotion containing a stronger dose of benzoyl peroxide. Other options include topical antibiotics or a retinoid (such as Retin A) designed to unclog pores. Very often treatment will involve a combination of these products. Because they can cause irritation during the first few weeks of use, Thellman-Karcher tells most patients to start by applying them every other night until their skin can tolerate more frequent applications.

Power pills. Because creams and lotions aren't always effective against stubborn breakouts, some patients move on to oral antibiotics. "This kills the bacteria that causes the inflammation that comes with some types of acne," says Thellman-Karcher. "It usually works quite well—sometimes permanently. But you often have to be on it for several months to see improvement."

Hormonal help. If your breakouts are especially bad right around your menstrual period, your doctor may prescribe certain oral contraceptives to keep your hormone levels steady throughout the month. Sometimes, this is enough to temper acne all by itself. Other times, birth control pills are prescribed in addition to other topical and oral treatments.

The last resort. If the above options are powerless against your pimples, your dermatologist may suggest Accutane, a very powerful drug that decreases oil production in the skin. While all acne treatments have side effects (consult with your doctor and read all labels carefully), Accutane comes with some especially serious ones, so it's reserved for the most stubborn, severe cases.

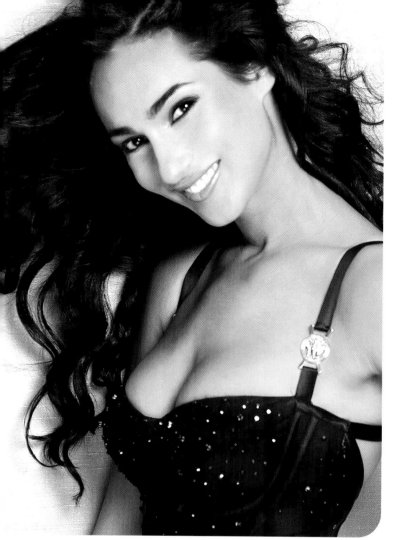

Asli Bayram, Germany, 2005 Miss Universe Contestant

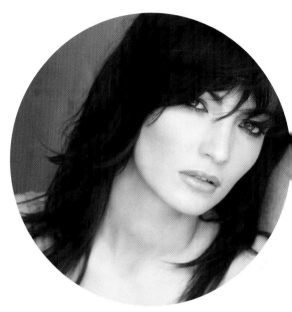

Mary Gormley, Ireland, 2005 Miss Universe Contestant

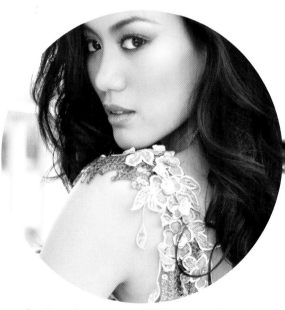

Chananporn Rosjan, Thailand, 2005 Miss Universe Contestant

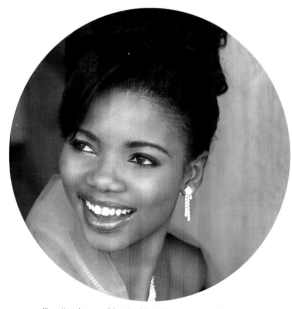

Roseline Amusu, Nigeria, 2005 Miss Universe Contestant

# great skin is the same in any language

Imagine how dull the world would be if skin came in only one shade or type. Year after year, the Miss Universe competition has offered the world a visual buffet of glowing, radiant complexions—from olive to chocolate to fair and freckled.

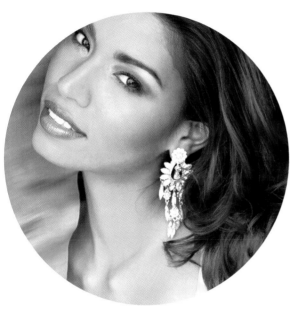

Sharita Sopacua, Netherlands, 2005 Miss Universe Contestant

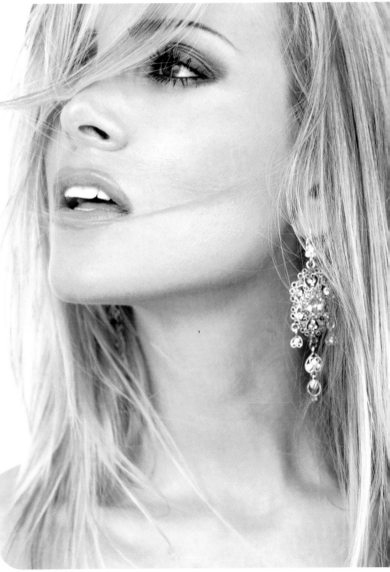

Jelena Mandic, Serbia & Montenegro, 2005 Miss Universe Contestant

49

# complexion quandary number 2: uneven pigmentation

Blotches and spots probably represent the second most common complaint Cheryl Thellman-Karcher hears from her pageant clientele—not to mention from scores of other women. Some have tiny red or bluish gray or brown spots left over from pimples that healed long before. Others have freckles or brown patches that have resulted from too much unprotected time in the sun. Almost always, this uneven pigmentation has taken years to develop. And thanks to modern technology, fading those errant patches of color—and sometimes erasing them entirely—requires far less time.

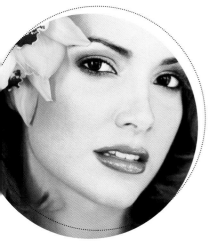

Denise M. Quiñones August
Puerto Rico, Miss Universe 2001

## know your enemy

Denise M Quiñones August (Puerto Rico, Miss Universe 2001) may not have to worry about blemishes, but for those who do, learning *why* those spots and blotches appear is the first step to kissing them goodbye.

### The acne's gone, but the memories linger on. When a pimple resolves itself, it tends to leave a calling card—in the form of a dark gray or brown spot. This hyperpigmentation can disappear within days or weeks, but it can stick around for much longer, depending on your skin type or tone. Post-acne marks in darker complexions (people of Asian, Latina, Indian, or African descent, for instance) usually take the longest to fade. And going outside without sunscreen while the mark is healing can make the waiting time even longer.

### Those beach vacations are written all over your face. That sun-kissed glow you get after being outside is actually sun-induced *injury* to the skin—which is why, after your tan fades, the skin is more freckled, mottled, and leathery than before. In the most extreme cases, that damage can result in skin cancer down the road.

### Your upper lip looks as if it has 5:00 shadow. You could have melasma, a patchy darkening of the skin, which typically occurs around the cheeks, forehead, bridge of nose, and upper lip. Melasma is most common in adult women—especially those of African, Indian, Asian, and Latina descent. It's a hereditary condition, but because hormonal changes can trigger it, pigmentation changes tend to occur with pregnancy or birth control use.

### You're seeing red, and it's not going away. Some skin conditions, such as rosacea, can cause capillaries to dilate—eventually resulting in permanent red blotches, especially around the nose and cheeks. This usually worsens with age, especially if you are frequently exposed to wind and extreme temperatures or if you drink a lot of alcohol.

# see spot run

Hardly anyone walks through life without accumulating some unwanted hyperpigmentation—not even Miss Universe. But if a pageant hopeful were to walk into Cheryl Thellman-Karcher's office today with an unwanted freckle, brown patch, or cluster of broken capillaries, she would have a wealth of treatment options. Here's a list of possibilities.

Sunscreen. A good facial sunscreen fights uneven pigmentation in two ways: First, it prevents spots from appearing in the first place by staving off damage from ultraviolet light. Second, it stops the sun from darkening existing marks. Again, sunscreen is especially important for those with Asian, African, Indian, or Latina complexions because darker skin types are more prone to hyperpigmentation. But dermatologists stress that everyone should slick on an SPF of at least 15 before going outside—whether running errands in town (even if the sky is overcast) or heading to the beach. Be sure to reapply for every two hours of sun exposure. For more information on sunscreen, turn to page 30.

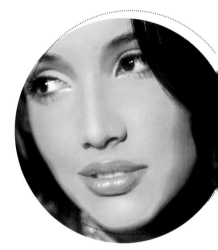

Amelia Vega, Dominican Republic
Miss Universe 2003

Antioxidants. Antioxidants, such as those occurring in green tea and vitamins E and C, may help mop up free radicals generated by sunlight. Left unchecked, free radicals can cause not only cancer but also freckles and age spots. Choose an antioxidant-containing sunscreen lotion. For more information on antioxidants, turn to page 53.

Topical fading products. There's a range of lotions and creams designed to brighten mottled or spotty skin. Creams containing alpha hydroxy acid may help some conditions, such as melasma, by sloughing off the top layers of the skin. Far more effective, however, are bleaching creams containing hydroquinone. Some combine bleach with retinoids designed to speed cell turnover. Topical fade treatments can take months of diligent use to show results. And because they can yield unpredictable results—especially on darker complexions—it's important to use them under a doctor's supervision.

Microdermabrasion. Basically a high-tech polishing device for the skin, microdermabrasion exfoliates the upper layers of the epidermis using a spray of aluminum-oxide crystals. After multiple sessions, spaced a few weeks apart, superficial spots may be less visible.

Lasers and light sources. If you have less time—and more money—to spend, certain lasers and other light-based treatments offer a speedy way to rid the skin of hyperpigmentation. Non-ablative lasers (which are less invasive) are relatively low-risk and come with few side effects (you can usually return to work the day after treatment). But they're typically less effective than ablative lasers, which work on the deeper layers of the skin. Just remember that the more powerful the laser, the higher the risk of scarring, as well as brown and white spots.

**universal truth** It may not make those freckles go away, but Barbara Palacios (Venezuela, Miss Universe 1986) swears her homemade exfoliation scrub boosts her skin's radiance: "I mix sugar with olive oil to create a paste and very gently scrub my face with it once a week," she says. This is best for dry, non-acne-prone skin types.

# complexion quandary number 3: aging skin

"I love being thirty-eight," says Angela Visser (Holland, Miss Universe 1989), who isn't the least bit daunted by the prospect of getting older. In fact, her favorite beauty and fashion icons are women who embrace their age, rather than fighting every fine line and wrinkle. Easy for Angela to say—this new mother still looks just as fabulously radiant as the day she won the crown. Most of us opt for a more proactive approach when it comes to handling the visible signs of aging. The first step to being proactive: Be prepared.

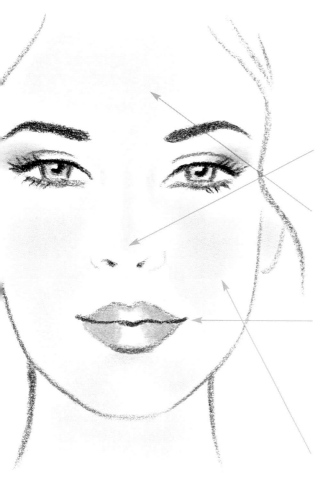

## a wrinkle in time

It may not be fair, but it's reality. The start of the skin's natural aging process starts after you leave your teen years, when the cell turnover begins to slow slightly and fat and collagen start to decrease.

Hyperpigmentation. Those brown spots and red blotches mentioned earlier tend to increase with age—in large part because of years of accumulated sun damage and decreased cell turnover.

Dryness. Your skin produces less oil as you get older—especially during and after menopause. That means, even if you spent your twenties mopping at your shiny nose, twenty years later your face may feel flaky and taut. This lack of natural moisture can make the skin appear papery and less supple.

Wrinkles and fine lines. Production of collagen and elastin slows dramatically as you age. This decreases the elasticity of the skin, along with its ability to bounce back from routine stretches and movements. Repeated motions such as squinting and smiling begin to translate into fine lines and wrinkles.

Fat loss. Anywhere else on the body, this would be a good thing. But the natural facial fat loss that occurs with age not only makes the hollows of the cheeks more apparent, but causes an overall sagging that extends all the way down to the neck.

# turning back the clock

The average Miss Universe isn't much older than a college grad—which means she's still blissfully unaware of the myriad antiaging treatments on the market these days. Here's a crash course in the latest and greatest.

From the tube. Topical treatments are the least-invasive line of attack against the visible signs of aging. Many of the creams and lotions used to fight hyperpigmentation (see page 51) can also serve to smooth texture and fine lines. Sunscreen, for instance, offers a preemptive strike by filtering out the UV rays that cause premature aging. Some research shows that creams containing copper and peptides can help decrease fine lines and prevent future ones. To lift away the top layers of the skin and reveal the smoother ones underneath, some doctors advise a gentle alpha hydroxy acid toner. Retinoids (such as Renova, Tazorac, and over-the-counter products containing retinol) provide much stronger exfoliation of the skin's upper layers—and also stimulate collagen production. Just remember that retinoids and retinol increase the skin's sensitivity to the sun. That means you should always apply them at bedtime and be especially diligent about slathering on sunscreen during the day.

From the chem lab. Chemical peels remove the top layer of the skin cells to reveal fresh, younger-looking skin below. To smooth fine lines and reduce age spots, most dermatologists use a solution of glycolic acid, lactic acid or salicylic acid. The deepest peels carry the most risk and downtime—but, when done successfully, erase the most damage. Superficial peels have minimal risk but require several treatments before showing significant improvement. That said, any peel (even mild, over-the-counter versions) will impart an immediate glow and rosiness to the skin, assuming you're not sensitive to the ingredients. Be sure to do a patch test first.

From the syringe. For more stubborn wrinkles and lines—and if you want to see immediate improvement—injectables offer a fast, effective fix. By far, one of the most popular is Botox (*Botulinum toxin*), which reduces the activity of the muscles responsible for wrinkles. It's best used in the upper portion of the face—the forehead and between the eyes, for example. An alternative or adjunct treatment to Botox is soft-tissue fillers, such as collagen and hyaluronic acid. The spongiest ones are quite good at plumping the lips, which tend to shrivel with age. And increasingly, women are using fillers of all kinds to smooth both deep wrinkles (such as those extending from the nostrils to the outer corners of the mouth) and finer ones (such as smile lines). Keep in mind that every injectable has a specific projected longevity. Discuss all the options and risks with your doctor.

# the art of aging gracefully

Wrinkles, schminkles! Miss Universe titleholders seem to have a knack for retaining their beauty as the years go by. In this 2005 photograph, Sylvia Hitchcock Carson (USA, Miss Universe 1967) and Margaret Gardiner (South Africa, Miss Universe 1978) prove that age truly is a state of mind.

## in her own words

"If I ran around in very demure clothing, that would put me in an older category immediately. I don't believe in stuffiness at any age—it's always better to look real. I've had people say to me that I'm prettier now than on the day I won the pageant."

—Sylvia Hitchcock Carson, USA, Miss Universe 1967

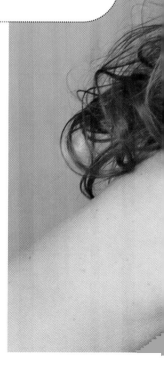

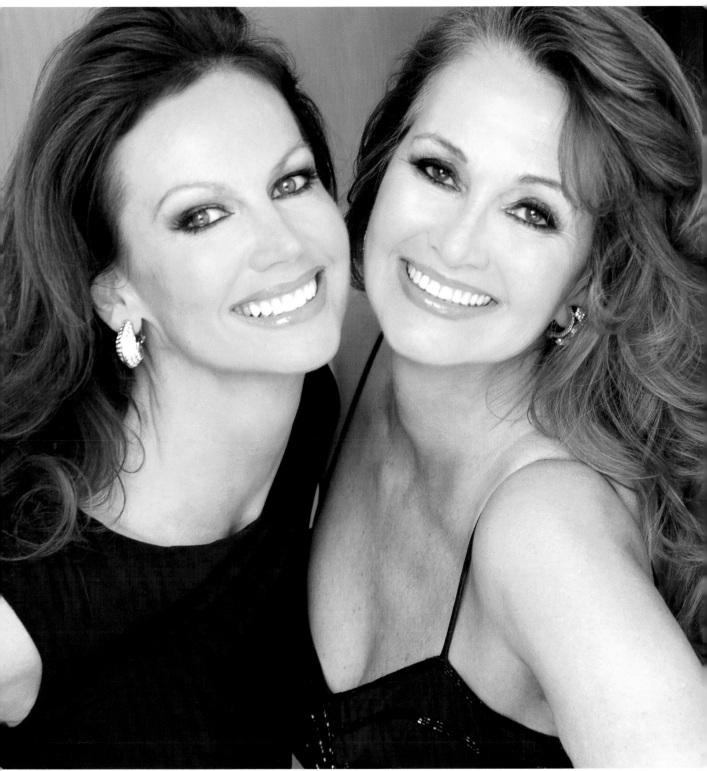

*Left:* Margaret Gardiner, South Africa, Miss Universe 1978
*Right:* Sylvia Hitchcock Carson, USA, Miss Universe 1967

# skin salvation in a bottle

Evening out the skin's texture and pigmentation is easier than ever, thanks to the slew of dream creams, lasers, and injectables available. But don't forget about the original skin perfecter: makeup. A good foundation and powder can make skin tone look more uniform, fade blemishes and scars, and even minimize the appearance of fine lines and wrinkles. No dermatologist appointment—or fat wallet—required.

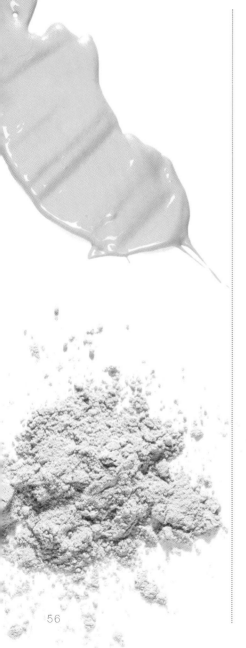

## the formula for success

Department store and drugstore shelves are lined with a dizzying array of foundations, powders, and concealers, each promising to make skin look absolutely flawless. We're not going to lie to you: Few makeups will completely erase *every* blemish and blotch—and the ones that can are usually too heavy for everyday use. "Ideal foundations don't mask skin," says CoverGirl makeup artist B.J. Gillian, who works on current and aspiring Miss Universes, Miss USAs, and Miss Teen USAs. "They blend into the skin." CoverGirl Advanced Radiance Age-Defying Compact Foundation and the TruBlend line of foundations and powders are all great choices. Here's how to find your perfect formula.

## the foundations

Tinted moisturizer. The current emphasis is on taking care of the skin—then covering it as little as possible. That's why tinted moisturizers are fast becoming a favorite alternative to true foundations. The caveat: Because they deliver a very sheer wash of color, tinted moisturizers are best for evening out relatively clear skin, not for camouflaging any serious imperfections.

Liquid foundation. Usually sheer or translucent, liquid foundation comes in a variety of weights. The more watery formulas offer slightly more coverage than a tinted moisturizer, without feeling the least bit heavy on the skin. They're also usually oil-free, which makes them a great choice if you're acne-prone. Thicker formulas can mute the appearance of blemishes, especially if topped with a bit of powder.

Cream foundation. Packed in jars or compacts, cream foundations offer thick, rich coverage—typically enough to hide scars, red patches, and obvious pimples. Ironically, however, if you have breakouts serious enough to warrant such heavy coverage, you should probably avoid most heavy foundations because of their tendency to clog pores. If you're acne-prone, stick to oil-free foundations that contain an anti-pimple medication such as salicylic acid.

Dual-finish foundation. This compact dual-finish foundation goes on creamy, then dries to a powder. The advantage of these formulas: the velvety, matte finish they'll give your complexion. If you have dry, flaky skin, avoid dual-finish makeup because it can make skin look chalky.

# the powders

Powder can be used instead of foundation—or on top of it. The best ones come in two basic formulations: loose and pressed.

Loose powder. Loose powder's big claim to fame: It feels weightless on the skin while leaving a soft, polished finish behind. Choose pigmented versions that match your skin or sheer translucent, which contains minimal pigment. Most makeup artists set foundation with a light dusting of loose powder to lock makeup in place and prevent shine.

Pressed powder. Pressed powder comes in a compact and offers a heavier, more finished coverage than loose powder—not to mention more staying power. Because of this, many women use it instead of foundation—making sure to touch up shiny areas, such as the T-zone, throughout the day.

# the concealers

Liquid concealer. Liquid concealers usually come in a jar and offer just slightly more coverage than an ordinary foundation. They are typically applied with a wand.

Creamy concealer. Generally sold in a tube, creamy concealers give a richer and fairly opaque look.

Cakey concealer. Cakey concealers tend to come in palettes or pots. Their pasty consistency grips the skin and remains in place, making them ideal for textured areas, such as scars.

Colored concealer. Colored concealers are made in a variety of formulations; these come in shades such as pink, green, and orange. While many experts swear by their ability to neutralize any skin discoloration under the sun (green supposedly neutralizes red), they can be risky if you don't know what you're doing. Best to stick to a skin-toned concealer (or one that's a shade above your natural skin tone) if you're at all skittish.

# ready, set, glow!

When Maritza Sayalero (Venezuela, Miss Universe 1979) was competing for the crown, it wasn't uncommon to "perfect" the skin using a pasty blend of makeup powder and water. Thankfully, a lot has changed since then. Nowadays, you know you've applied your base properly if nobody knows you're wearing it. Here are five steps to a beautiful base.

Maritza Sayalero
Venezuela, Miss Universe 1979

1. Cleanse the face. Wash with a mild cleanser. Because foundation and powder tend to magnify flakes, use a gentle exfoliating scrub over any dry patches.

2. Pat dry. Blot the face with a clean towel, then slick an oil-free moisturizer (or a richer cream if skin is very dry) over parched or rough areas. If you're using a tinted moisturizer instead of foundation, apply a coat all over the face, and proceed to step four.

3. Lay your foundation. Allow any moisturizer to soak into the skin for five minutes. Then, using a clean makeup sponge, dot foundation on the eyelids, nose, and center of the cheeks. Blend the formula over the face (don't forget under the eyes) with your sponge until the makeup is no longer visible on the skin. If using pressed powder instead of foundation, apply it to the entire face—or only in spots that require coverage.

4. Disguise the extras. Apply skin-toned concealer over blemishes, and blend until concealer is no longer visible.

5. Take a powder. For an added finish—or to stave off excess shine—dust over the foundation with translucent loose powder.

# just add color

No self-respecting Miss Universe contestant would think of stepping on stage without a pop of vibrant red or pink on her cheeks. Wearing quite that much color doesn't fly in real life, but there's not a woman out there who couldn't benefit from a shot of blush or bronzer—and even a touch of highlighter.

Blushes. Blushes come in powders, creams, and gels. If you're already wearing loose powder, you have no choice but to go with a powder blush. (Or else end up with a pasty face.) Powder blush is easy to apply and will stay on the face the longest. Cream blush is best for dry skin and doesn't cling well to oilier complexions. Gels offer a sheer shot of color, and blend easily into the skin, making it look as if the color is radiating from within.

Bronzers. You'll find bronzers in powders and creams, both of which add a soft, tawny glow to the skin. The blush rules above apply to bronzers as well: If you're wearing powder, use a powder bronzer; choose a bronzer cream if you have a cream foundation. Bronzers come in a variety of colors, but the best one for you is usually a couple of shades darker than your natural complexion. They look most natural when worn during the summer or early fall.

Highlighters. Highlighters are creams and powders with an ever-so-slight sheen. (Avoid ones that visibly sparkle on the skin.) Dabbed over blush or bronzer, they're designed to add a slight glow to the face—*not* an allover shine. The key to using highlighters is to hold back on the application.

## universal truth

The latest crop of blushes is so sheer that most women can get away with wearing virtually any shade under the sun. As a general rule, however, those with cooler skin tones look best in rosy pinks and berries. Olive complexions are most flattered with apricots and rusty reds.

Applied correctly, blush and bronzer can enliven and warm up the face. Done wrong, that added color can look suspiciously like a fever rash. For those who prefer the former approach, we've mapped it out for you. Note that the illustrations are exaggerated to show placement.

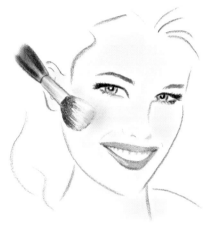

Smile into the mirror so that the apples of the cheeks are visible. If wearing a powder blush, brush color over the apples. Then blend the remaining color on the brush up toward the ears. If wearing a cream or gel blush, use a sponge or your fingers to swirl color over the apples, then pat whatever is remaining up toward your ears. Finish with a bit of highlighter applied along the tops of your cheekbones.

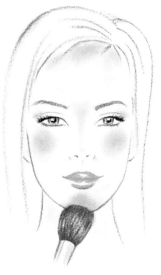

Blend for a natural look.

Apply bronzer wherever the sun would naturally hit, using either a large, fluffy brush or your fingertips. The best spots are the tops of your cheekbones, the top center of your forehead (close to the hairline), the chin, and the bridge of your nose.

# tool box

Preventing, repairing, and hiding skin imperfections is a piece of cake—provided you're armed with the proper equipment.

### Blush and bronzer.
Choose one subtle shade of blush and bronzer for daytime and one that looks slightly more dramatic, for evening.

### Brushes.
Your kit should include two large, natural-bristle brushes for blush/ bronzer and loose powder application; a small, flat-tipped brush and a pointier one for concealer; and a pack of clean sponges for swabbing on foundation.

### Cleanser.
Find a cleanser you (and your dermatologist) love—but don't be afraid to reassess it six months later. Skin that seems impossibly oily during the summer can turn parched and tight come December.

### Foundation and powder.
To find precisely the right shade for you, test three different colors of foundation and powder along your jaw-line—not on the back of your hand, which is often darker than your face. To find your perfect match without opening the package, hold the bottle against the upper part of your chin.

### Highlighter.
Remember to use a highlighter that adds a slight sheen to the skin—*not* sparkle.

### Moisturizer.
Unless your skin is very dry, start with an oil-free moisturizer. Lotions containing sunscreen are great, but because most of us tend to apply facial moisturizers sparingly, you'll probably want to keep a separate SPF product on hand for extended periods outside.

### Treatment products.
Discuss your problem issues with your dermatologist before selecting which products are best for you.

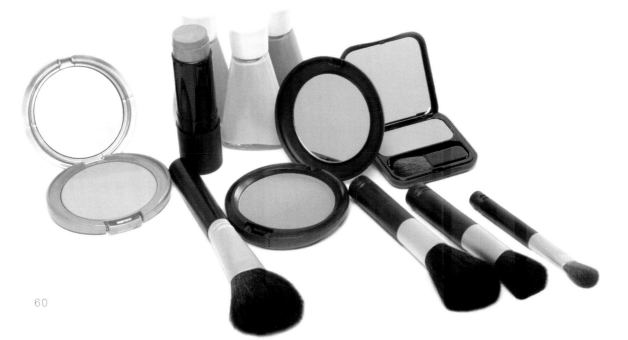

# how to cover just about anything

When there's no time or money for a laser appointment and your ordinary makeup just isn't doing the trick, it's concealer to the rescue! Finally, the cure for whatever facial blemish ails you.

**Acne scars.** Cover acne scars with a cakey concealer, filling in the center of the scar. For a raised scar, pat only the top with concealer. Finish by pressing loose powder over the area.

**Dark circles.** To conceal dark circles, first apply a speck of foundation using a damp sponge. Follow by pressing a creamy concealer onto the darkened areas with a small, flat brush. Pat with a clean, damp sponge, then use a puff to press loose powder over the concealer.

**Freckles and moles.** Don't expect to cover freckles and moles completely—and why would you want to? Instead, choose a foundation that dries to a powder finish. Using a puff, press the formula into the skin. To cover a more prominent mole, dot the top of it with a thick, opaque concealer. Rather than blending it, allow it to dry for a minute and set the concealer in place with a dab of compact foundation.

**Pimples.** Some experts advising minimizing the redness of pimples by soaking a cotton swab in Visine and putting it in the freezer for a minute. Then touch the swab to your blemish for thirty seconds, let dry, then dab a dot of cakey concealer on the top of the bump. Use a small, flat brush to blend the edges, allow concealer to dry, then add another layer if needed. Finish with a light pat of loose powder.

**Redness.** Apply your foundation as you normally would, then pat a thin coat of creamy concealer (try one that exactly matches your skin) onto the spots that are still red. Wait a few minutes for it to dry, then add another coat, and repeat the process until the redness is gone. Dust with loose powder to set the makeup.

# the mane event

## Wendy Fitzwilliam, Trinidad & Tobago, Miss Universe 1998

When a good friend begged Wendy Fitzwilliam to enter the Miss Trinidad & Tobago pageant nearly a decade ago, she was a budding law student—and far more preoccupied with books than beauty. "Pageants came across as very superficial with no promise or future," Wendy remembers. "But then my friend said, 'The worst that can happen is you'll win—and have a three-week vacation when you represent our country at the Miss Universe competition.'"

The worst happened—twice. Wendy took her country's crown, then jetted off to Hawaii where she charmed the Miss Universe judges. In retrospect, she notes that vying for the world title hardly qualified as a vacation. "I had a ball, but this was real work!" says Wendy. "I was determined to make the top ten. I try not to do anything at less than 100 percent."

These days, back in her native Trinidad, the brainy beauty still refuses to rest on her laurels. As an executive at a leading technology company, a Goodwill Ambassador to the United Nations, and chair of the Hibiscus Foundation, an organization she created to heighten AIDS awareness, Wendy remains firmly in the public eye. So when it comes to appearance, she can't afford to have so much as a hair out of place. And that's quite a feat in the steamy Caribbean, where temperatures regularly climb into the nineties and the average humidity hovers around 85 percent. Here's how to keep your tresses looking smooth, shiny, and fabulous all year round—and at any latitude.

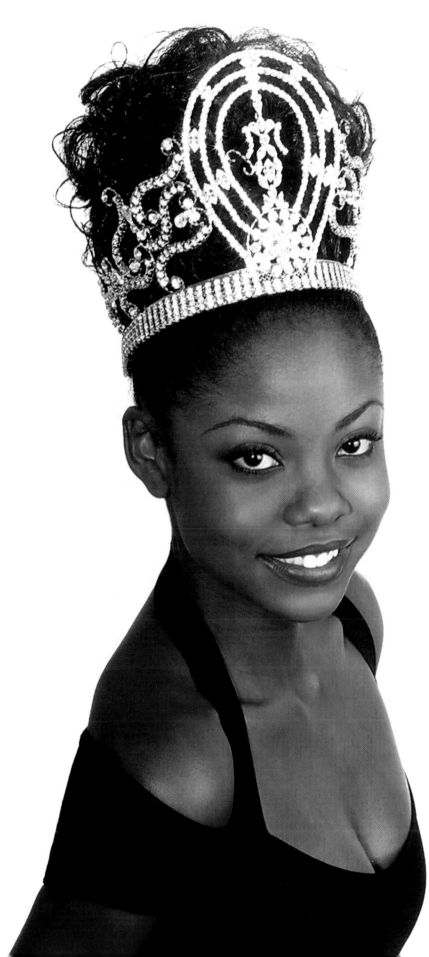

# starting fresh

Miss Universe hopefuls have an intimate relationship with hair sprays, mousses, and gels. Unfortunately, the same products that lock fragile updos in place for hours can leave a heavy, sticky residue behind if not properly washed out. The same goes for the milder silicone serums and curl creams many of us wear daily. The key to shiny, bouncy, healthy-looking hair: Cleanse just enough to keep dulling buildup at bay—then follow with a good conditioner to keep tresses from drying out. New York hairstylist John Barrett, who has been Miss Universe's mane man for years, reveals four ways to come clean.

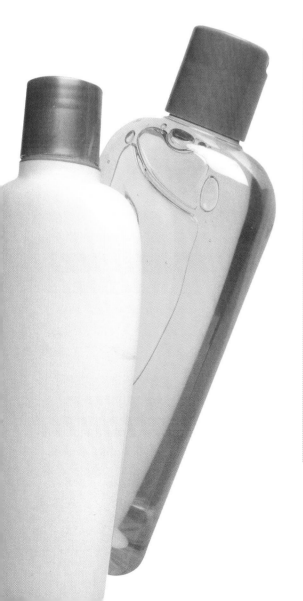

Scan the label. Choose shampoos and conditioners that complement your hair type. For those with fine or oily strands, "it's better to use a clear shampoo—one that doesn't say *cream* anywhere on the bottle—and a lightweight conditioner," says Barrett. If you have coarser, dry hair, look for shampoos designed to hydrate and conditioners containing jojoba, avocado, and nut or seed oils. And while women with normal hair can get away with using nearly any good-quality formulas, Barrett suggests boosting the shine by treating your hair with white vinegar once a month. "Just dilute two tablespoons in a little water and rinse it through your hair," he notes. "It will balance the pH, making the hair look extremely healthy."

Lather up. Massage a quarter-sized dollop of shampoo into your hair—making sure to include the scalp and the nape of the neck where dirt and oil tend to collect. Moving your fingers in small circular motions over the scalp will also increase blood flow, encouraging faster hair growth and bringing fresh, healthy oils to the surface for more luxurious locks.

To add a special luster to dry, coarse, unruly hair, first shampoo, condition, and rinse as usual—then try Barrett's trick: Just before turning off the shower, rub a tiny drop of conditioner between your palms, slick it over your locks, and leave it in. "This will help weigh down your hair and smooth out the frizz," he says.

Don't repeat. Because real life doesn't involve pageant-sized portions of super-hold hair spray, shampooing twice in one shower usually isn't necessary. In fact, Barrett suggests shampooing only once every other day, using only conditioner on off days to keep hair hydrated and manageable. "Ninety-five percent of people overwash their hair," he says. "This also goes for women with oily hair. Shampooing too often will overstimulate the scalp, causing it to produce more oil."

Condition correctly. Conditioner is essentially a moisturizer for your hair, filling in damaged areas of the hair shaft and sealing the cuticles flat so that tresses look smoother and feel more manageable. But even the best formula is only as effective as the application. To evenly coat every strand, first rub conditioner between your hands, then rake through the hair with your fingers, gently loosening tangles—or drag it through with a wide-tooth comb. Because the inch of hair closest to the scalp is usually oily, keep conditioner away from the roots. If you have very oily or limp locks, apply it only to the lower half of your hair. Regardless of what hair type you are, give a final rinse with cool water to help smooth the cuticles and boost shine.

# dirty little secret

John Barrett has executed so many crown-worthy updos that he could practically do a French twist or chignon in his sleep. One of his best secrets to flawless, elegant results every time? Don't wash your hair. "Slightly dirty hair is always easier to work with," he says. "It's more moldable and tends to stay in place." If you've already shampooed that morning, add a bit of faux grime to the hair by massaging in a touch of pomade.

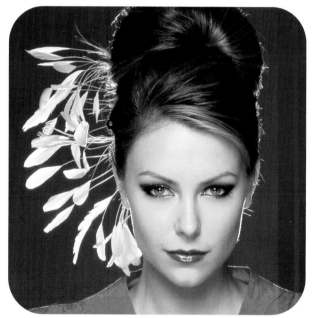

Jennifer Hawkins, Australia, Miss Universe 2004

## universal truth

Yvonne Agneta-Ryding (Sweden, Miss Universe 1984) admits that she often straightens her curly hair with a flat iron—but she counters the damage by putting her own spin on one of hairstylist John Barrett's favorite tips. Once a week, after shampooing and gently towel-drying her locks, she applies a hair mask designed for dry, thick hair, such as Kérastase Nutritive Masquintense. "Then I sit in the sauna for fifteen minutes, so that my hair gets warm," she says. Heat speeds penetration into the hair shaft and helps lock in conditioners for even silkier, softer results.

# damage control

Angela Visser (Holland, Miss Universe 1989) has a low-maintenance approach to hair care that doesn't leave room for blow-dryers, hot rollers, and straight irons. "I let it air-dry every day," she says. "The only time I used those tools was for Miss Universe–related events." And as any pageant contestant can attest, no woman is immune to the frying effects of blow-dryers, hot rollers, and straight irons. The trick is knowing how to minimize injury— and how to make ravaged hair look as good as new.

Don't play rough. Vigorously towel-drying after a shower can ruffle the hair cuticles and make locks harder to comb, resulting in more damage. The best way to deal with soaking-wet strands: Use that towel to blot dry.

Wear protective gear. Before bringing a hot styling tool anywhere near your head, use a spray or serum designed to guard against damage. Farouk BioSilk Silk Therapy's line of shampoos and styling products seal protective moisturizers into the hair when exposed to heat. And products containing silicone minimize damage by creating a shielding barrier between the tool and your tresses.

Save time, save your hair. For a safer blow-out, let the hair dry naturally until it's damp, then use the dryer to style the hair into shape. Set the temperature to medium (not hot), and hold the nozzle at least two inches from the hair.

Take a break. When not dashing from one fabulous event to the next, the world's crowned beauties put their feet up and give their locks a breather. "If I have time, I try to let my hair air-dry as much as possible," says Yvonne Agneta-Ryding (Sweden, Miss Universe 1984).

Feed your head. For those who have their manes teased, tousled, and tortured on an almost daily basis, John Barrett believes a deep-conditioning hair mask, used at least once a month, is essential. Unlike old-school formulas that came with ugly plastic caps, the latest versions (Barrett makes one called Bee Healed) are applied before bedtime and rinsed out in the morning. Mona Grudt (Norway, Miss Universe 1990) regularly uses either a deep treatment or her ordinary conditioner before going to sleep. "I put my hair in a bun, put a towel around my pillow, and rinse it out the next morning," she says. "The hair really gets its shine back and looks alive again."

Disguise the damage. Silicone creams, sprays, and serums can effectively hide breaks and splits in the hair—provided you use them correctly. Because overdosing will weigh down the hair, apply only a few drops to the ends or to select frizzy patches. One warning: Silicone is especially guilty of leaving a dulling residue behind, so regular users should wash hair with a clarifying shampoo at least every other night to keep buildup at bay.

Cut it out. If even the silkiest conditioners and styling creams won't resuscitate your frazzled split ends, take the hint and get rid of them. "Some people feel that it's better to have long pieces of dry, burned hair than healthy shorter hair," says Barrett, who advises scheduling regular trims every six to eight weeks. "Taking just an eighth of an inch off can make all the difference."

# making the cut

There's certainly no law stating which haircuts best flatter which face shape, but we'd like to suggest some guidelines.

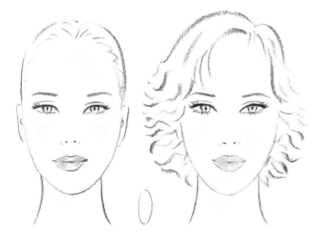

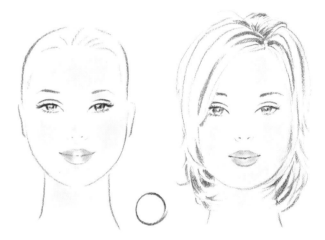

### If Your Face Is Oval

Choose almost any cut you want—but keep in mind that very long or very short styles may accentuate a long face. To create the illusion of more width, cut bangs (if hair is straight) or enhance natural waves (if hair is curly) with a diffusing blow-dryer and curling cream. A chin-length bob will also add fullness.

### If Your Face Is Round

Choose a cut that hangs below the chin—or a very short style with tapered layers. Either way, wispy pieces that fall softly around the cheeks and chin will de-emphasize fullness. Parting the hair on the side and styling height into the crown of the head can add length to the face.

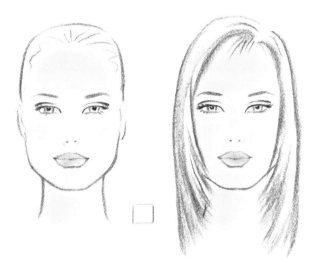

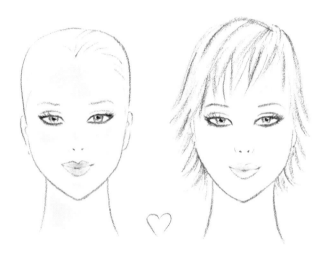

## If Your Face Is Square

Choose face-framing cuts to counter the harshness of the chin and jaw-line. If hair is long, that means snipping layers so that they start at the jaw and gradually get longer toward the back. If you're going short, ask for a choppy, pixie style. And avoid anything blunt, including squared-off bobs or straight-across bangs.

## If Your Face Is Heart-Shaped

Choose either a thick, choppy pixie cut that's full on top or a longer style with layers that start at the cheekbones and graduate downward. If you have bangs, they're best worn brushed off to one side.

# tint condition

The right hair color can do far more than make a so-so mane look spectacular. It can create the illusion of clearer skin and a brighter smile—and can take years off your age. And these days, Miss Universe is demonstrating that better than just about anyone. Rather than automatically choosing, say, a bright platinum blond color, the world's crowned beauties are letting their skin tone be their guide—with dazzling results. "The look is more muted than it was in the past, but still very striking," says William Howe, colorist at New York City's John Barrett Salon, who has been tending to titleholders' locks since 2000. "It's a softer look—and it's also more feminine."

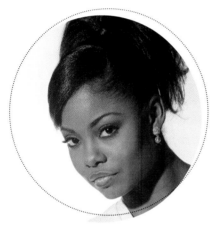

Wendy Fitzwilliam, Trinidad & Tobago
Miss Universe 1998

## warm complexion
(golden, olive, or brown skin)

The goal: Counteract the skin's sallow tones and keep hair from looking too harsh against the face.

The unbeatable brunette: Chocolate browns

The bodacious blonde: Soft, golden mixed with caramel

The most ravishing red: Dark auburn and cinnamon hues

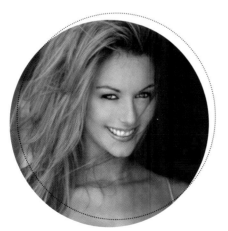

Jennifer Hawkins, Australia
Miss Universe 2004

## cool complexion
(fair skin, often with blue or green eyes)

The goal: Make the skin look creamier and less ruddy.

The unbeatable brunette: Ashy browns

The bodacious blonde: Champagne and beige tones

The most ravishing red: Bright red or burgundy shades

# universal truth 👑

It sounds counterintuitive, but when it comes to hair color, attaining a truly natural look usually requires *more* time in the salon. The secret behind the "I was born with it" blond hue of Yvonne Agneta-Ryding (Sweden, Miss Universe 1984): Combine several similar shades rather than going with a flat monochromatic tint. "I use three colors," she says. "The first is a little darker than my natural color, the second is a warm, light reddish, and the third is very blond." Other shade combinations that are flattering on nearly everyone: chocolate-brown base with caramel highlights or a light red base flecked with soft golden streaks.

# highlight placement

Howe doesn't see much harm in using home hair color kits for single-process jobs—as long as you're only altering the hair by one or two shades. But double-process highlighting generally requires the skilled hands and eyes of a professional. (At the very least, you need someone who can see the back of your head!) Most colorists still create highlights by isolating bleached pieces of hair with foils. But Howe prefers the baliage technique, painting highlights directly onto the hair without foils. This method involves more artistry, but done right, it creates a look that's slightly haphazard and very natural looking. And because bleach is allowed to bleed slightly from the highlighted pieces onto the rest of the head, you end up with no harsh lines of demarcation—and a less obvious growing-out period.

When it comes to placement, "I'm not a big fan of anything that's too even or symmetrical," says Howe. To borrow a cliché, the key to good hair color is location, location, location.

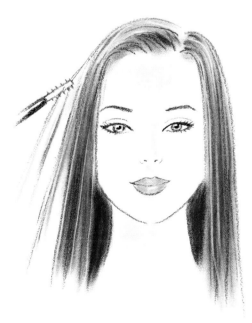

# operation preservation

Faded, washed-out highlights can make even the prettiest pageant crown look downright dingy. Howe advises clients to have their color touched up every four to twelve weeks—the farther you are from your natural color, the more frequently you should visit the salon. Between appointments, here's how the most stunning women in the world keep their color truer, longer.

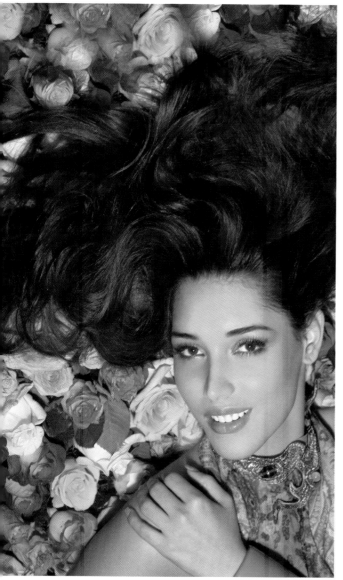

Amelia Vega, Dominican Republic, Miss Universe 2003

**Get a little dirty.** Cutting back to two or three shampoos per week not only keeps your hair from drying out, it saves your color.

**Choose the right formulas.** When you do lather up, use a shampoo and conditioner designed for color-treated hair. Two of Howe's favorite lines: Phytologie, Biolage, and L'Oréal Color Vive.

**Rinse out the bad stuff.** Rinse your hair as soon as you step out of the ocean or pool. "Salt water acts as an acid that strips color, and chlorine is a killer on blondes—I've had many clients come back from summer vacation with green hair," warns Howe.

**Protect yourself.** If sun can fade your living room couch, just think of what it'll do to your $300 highlights. In fact, Howe often takes his blonde, sun-worshipping clients down a few shades just before summer to keep their hair from looking too pale by Labor Day. To protect any shade from sun fade, slick conditioner (preferably one containing UV filters) over damp hair before exposing it to the rays. Or better yet, shelter it all under a wide-brimmed hat or scarf.

## universal truth ♛

If you absolutely can't get to the salon (and are in dire need of a touchup), Howe insists there's nothing wrong with a little cheating. He suggests buying a home coloring kit in a shade that most closely matches your base color and dabbing it on your roots with a cotton ball or Q-tip.

# chasing the grays away

For women blessed with naturally stunning color, finding those first few grays is enough to make them want to dive into a vat of hair dye. They'd be wise to reconsider. Most graying starts in one area (often around the temples), so it's usually possible to spot-color the affected portion and leave the rest of the head alone. Those trying this at home should choose a tint one shade up from their natural one. "It's better to err on the lighter side than on the darker side, especially when you're dealing with the hair around your face," says Howe, who advises using a semipermanent color.

For women who have gray scattered throughout the hair, a trip to the colorist is probably a good idea. "Most of us lose pigment in the skin as we age, so an expert will know whether you should go up a shade or two to compensate," Howe notes. "For someone who is forty-five and has a handful of gray hairs, she can probably stay with her base shade and ask for some beautiful golden highlights. If she's 80 percent gray, her skin tone may have changed enough to require lightening the base shade as well."

# style evolution

Aside from her trademark Mikimoto headpiece, Miss Universe's hair has always been her crowning glory. Here's a look back at how the international beauties have backcombed, ironed, and hot-rolled their way to the top.

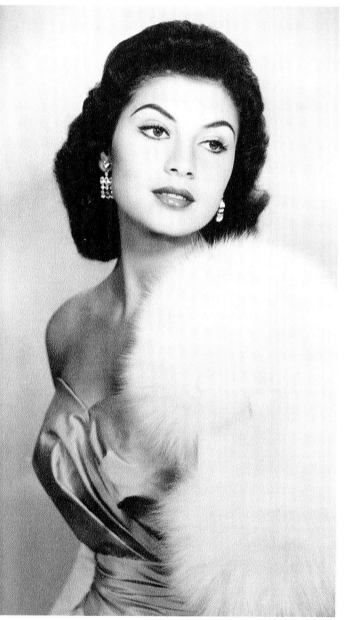

Gladys Zender, Peru, Miss Universe 1957

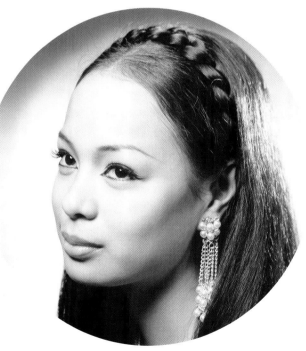

Gloria Diaz, Philippines, Miss Universe 1969

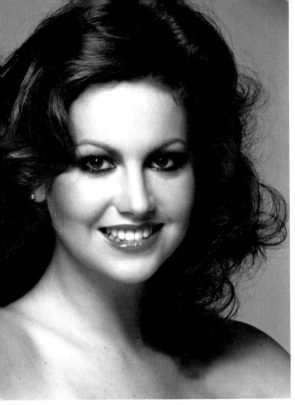

Margaret Gardiner, South Africa, Miss Universe 1978

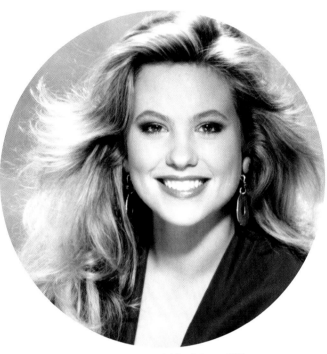

Angela Visser, Holland, Miss Universe 1989

Natalie Glebova, Canada, Miss Universe 2005

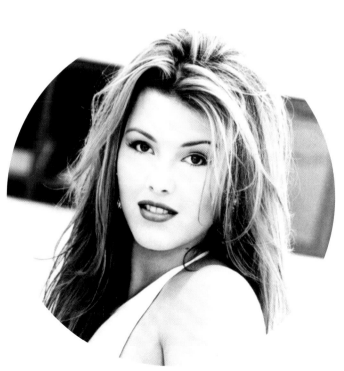

Alicia Machado, Venezuela, Miss Universe 1996

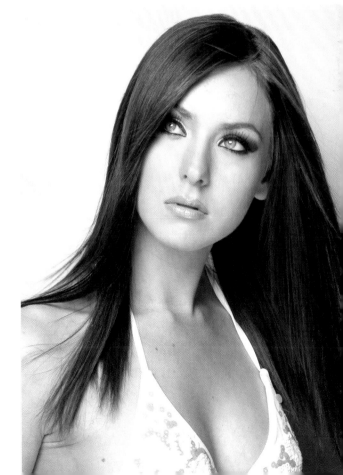

# tool box

When Maritza Sayalero (Venezuela) was vying for the Miss Universe title in 1979, she had to borrow a curling iron from her roommate, Miss Colombia. Shortly after her win, she bought one of her own—not to mention a set of hot rollers and a hair-dryer with a comb. Twenty-five years later, when it comes to standing out from the competition, owning the right tools is everything.

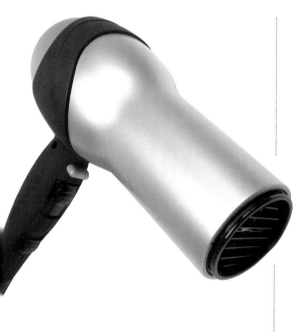

Blow-dryer. Power is everything, so look for a dryer with 1,500 to 1,875 watts. (The thicker the hair, the more wattage required.) Diehard blow-dryer fans should consider investing in a few bells and whistles: A cold setting can add shine when blasted over the hair during the final minutes of styling. A nozzle attachment effectively directs the flow of air—very helpful for straightening. A diffuser scatters the air, an essential feature for defining bouncy curls. Finally, ionic dryers shrink water droplets on the hair, reducing drying time.

Brushes. "One great brush that every model and Miss Universe owns is the Mason Pearson," says New York hairstylist John Barrett. Its bristles offer a combination of natural boar (for shine) and nylon (for control). "It's great for keeping hair very smooth. When I'm styling hair that looks dry, I rub a drop of baby oil between my palms, slick it over the hair, and brush it through with the Mason Pearson." Those who regularly blow out their locks (see page 83) should also buy a large boar bristle round brush.

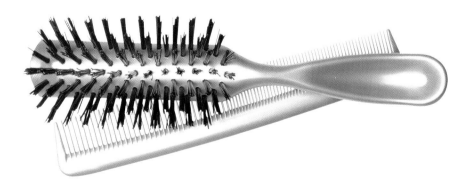

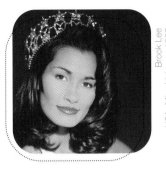

## in her own words

●●●●●

"Believe it or not, I don't even own a hairbrush. My thick, Korean hair kind of does its own thing. If I want it to look really bouncy, I'll smash it all on top of my head in a ponytail bun to dry, then rip it down right before I leave the house and just run my hands through it for waves."

— Brook Lee, USA, Miss Universe 1997

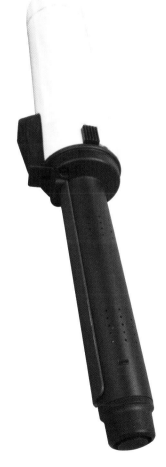

**Curling iron.** Whether you have ringlets or bone-straight hair, a curling iron is invaluable. Turn unruly locks into big, smooth waves by holding a large-barrel curling iron (over an inch in diameter) horizontally and rolling three-inch sections up toward the roots. To coax curls out of flatter hair, hold a three-quarter-inch curling iron vertically and twist smaller sections around it.

**Flat iron.** Barrett calls the flat iron "one of the magic of tools—one that every woman should have on her dressing table." These wonders come in a variety of shapes and sizes, but his favorites are narrow and small—better to maneuver through thick, unruly hair. And while some models are designed to be used on wet hair, Barrett advises waiting until locks are fully dry to avoid damaging them.

# african hair

Like many Trinidadians, Wendy Fitzwilliam has some African ancestry, which means her tresses demand tender loving care. "It's a running joke that black women obsess about their hair," says Wendy. "We do to some extent, but that's because it's just not as versatile in its natural state as Caucasian or Asian hair." Because Wendy typically likes to go flowing and straight, she has her hair chemically straightened or relaxed once every eight weeks, by the same seasoned professional she's been seeing for years. "My hair is very fine, so to keep it from drying out, I'll only trust stylists who are great at applying chemicals to black hair," she says. Here are four more ways Wendy keeps her mane in shape.

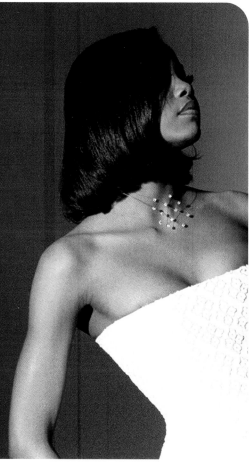

Wendy Fitzwilliam, Trinidad & Tobago, Miss Universe 1998

Cleanse with care. Relaxer can damage hair, decreasing its ability to retain moisture. Because shampoos strip away natural oils, Wendy has her hair washed at the salon once a week at the most.

Limit harsh styling. Because blow-drying and setting hair can zap the life out of it, Wendy does these sparingly—only after those once-a-week shampoos. For the first three days after her professional blow-set, she says, "All I have to do is finger comb my hair into place in the mornings. After that, I pull it back for the rest of the week or curl the ends with a curling iron."

Restore moisture. Wendy's desert-island product for keeping her tresses hydrated: "Hair grease," she says. "I just put a little bit on my fingertips and apply it to my scalp. One container usually lasts me a year." (Check out the hair care aisle in most drugstores for this pomade-like product, which usually contains mineral oil.) Then, after combing her locks into shape, she boosts its sheen with Aveda Brilliant Spray-on Shine. "I spray a little on my hands and rub it over the surface of my hair."

Think deep. To keep hair looking sleek and supple over the long term, Wendy says regular deep conditioning (use a treatment containing natural oils such as avocado or shea butter) is an absolute necessity. "It's *very* important for black women," she says. "I have a treatment every two weeks."

Yvonne Agneta-Ryding was fortunate to have the kind of hair that dries naturally into a pile of soft curls. For those without big-time volume programmed into their DNA, here's a lesson in body building.

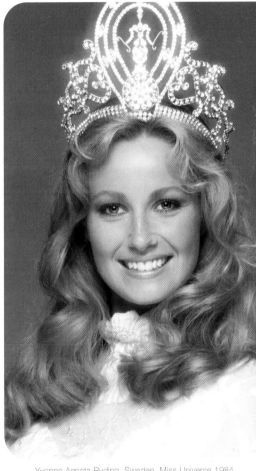

Yvonne Agneta-Ryding, Sweden, Miss Universe 1984

**Wash well.** Heavy buildup can make fine hair look even more so. For an instant volume boost, use a clear shampoo, which cleans away residue far better than the creamy kind. Follow with a lightweight rinse-out conditioner or a spray leave-in version applied only to the ends of the hair. (Steer clear of conditioners with words such as *rich, repair,* or *deep* on the bottle.)

**Pump up the volume.** Spritz locks with volumizing spray, paying special attention to the roots, then scrunch with your fingers to encourage waves.

**Diffuse the situation.** If not air-drying the hair, use a blow-dryer with a diffuser attachment on medium setting. Rather than scrunching the hair further, cup the hair in the palm of your hand as you direct air over it for a minute, then do the same with another section. When the hair is halfway dry, hold your head upside down and continue until the hair is almost completely dry. Raise your head up and gently finger-comb tresses into place.

**Take a booster shot.** If your mane starts to fall midday, either mist lightly with water and scrunch hair into place, or pile the hair into a ponytail on the top of your head for twenty to thirty minutes and spritz the roots with a bit more volumizing spray.

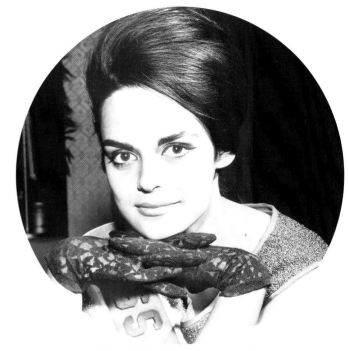

Corinna Tsopei, Greece, Miss Universe 1964

Irene Saez, Venezuela, Miss Universe 198

Akiko Kojima, Japan, Miss Universe 1959

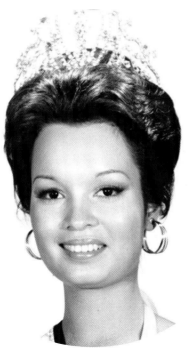

Margarita Moran, Philippines, Miss Universe 1973

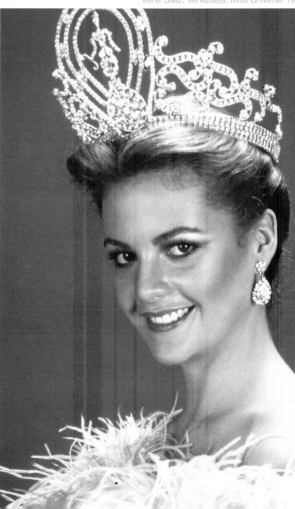

A well-crafted updo flatters far more than just the hair. It can give a little lift to the face, add drama and polish to an ordinary black dress, and make a so-so neck look positively swanlike. It's no wonder women from all over the world choose the classic chignon or French twist year after year when competing for the Miss Universe title. Today's updos may be a bit looser and more creative than those of decades past—but they're every bit as graceful.

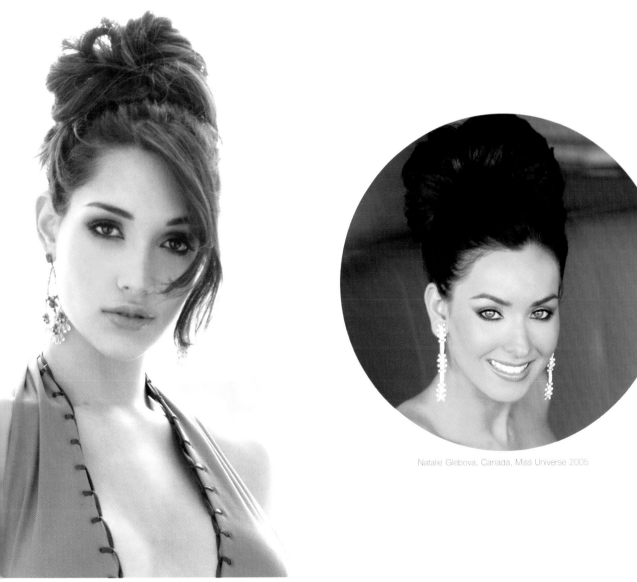

Natalie Glebova, Canada, Miss Universe 2005

# john's very doable 'do

He may execute some rather elaborate updos for his crown-wearing clients, but John Barrett says one of his favorite styles is embarrassingly simple.

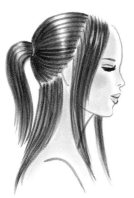 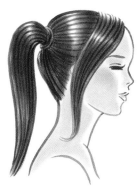 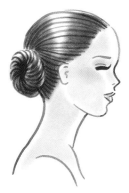 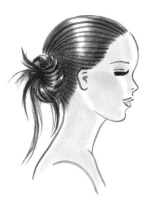

1. Using an elastic band, secure a tight ponytail, using the middle third of your hair from the crown to an inch above the nape of the neck. (Leave one-third of your hair hanging at the neck and one-third loose between the crown and the forehead.)

2. Take the hair hanging at the nape, smooth it with a brush and a dab of silicone serum, and wrap it around the top of the ponytail, securing it against the head with a hairpin. Smooth the loose section of hair between the crown and forehead, and part it on the side so that you have two sections.

3. Wrap one section under the base of the ponytail, securing it sleekly against the head with a pin, then do the same with the other section. Wind the ponytail around itself to form a smooth bun.

4. For a funkier look, tease out the tail.

## universal truth

To protect her fine, delicate hair from the ravages of the blow-dryer, Maritza Sayalero (Venezuela, Miss Universe 1979) coats her locks with Matrix Biolage Fortifying Heat Styler. This infuses hair strands with strengthening proteins when exposed to hot tools.

# the sleek story

Even as more and more crown-bound women are embracing their natural hair textures, plenty continue to blow-dry their natural curls and waves into smooth submission. Barrett shows us how it's done.

**Prepare.** After blotting the hair dry with a towel, lightly coat strands with a styling product: mousse for soft hold or gel for sleeker, stronger hold. Save any silicone serums until the end.

**Relax.** Rather than reaching for the blow-dryer the minute you step out of the shower, let the hair air-dry for a bit first. "One of the biggest mistakes women make is starting when hair is too wet—you'll just get tired and fed up by the end," he says. Instead, chill out and wait until tresses are only damp before cranking up the hot air.

**Prioritize.** "If the hairline is blown out beautifully, you can get away with the rest of the hair being a little less than great," confides Barrett. If you have bangs, start by combing them forward and holding them tightly with your fingers as you blow them dry, directing the nozzle starting from the roots. "Do the same for the entire hairline," he says. "Then lightly run a brush over it once the hair is dry."

**Divide and conquer.** Separate the hair into four or five clean sections, detangling each with a wide-tooth comb before clipping all but one of them to the head. Blow-dry the loose section, pulling it taut toward the floor with a large round brush and rolling it either under or out at the ends. Keep the blow-dryer's nozzle a few inches from the brush at all times, directing it down to the floor to keep the cuticles flat and smooth. Repeat with the other sections, rolling some under and flipping some out at the ends so that the hair doesn't look too uniform.

**Bring out the big guns.** Flat irons and rollers let you cheat your way to Miss Universe-caliber polish in minutes. To use a flat iron, Barrett presses small sections of completely dried hair, starting at the roots and working his way down to the ends. Or for smooth, sultry waves, he winds nearly dried hair in large Velcro rollers and pins them against the head before blasting them with the blow-dryer to set them. After a few minutes, he removes the rollers and gently tousles the hair with his hands.

**Seal the deal.** Silicone serums and creams can impart healthy shine to hair that's prone to frizz or plagued by split ends—just don't use more than a drop or two. "It should be used sparingly and only on the ends after you've completed styling," says Barrett. "If you use too much, it can make the hair look very slimy."

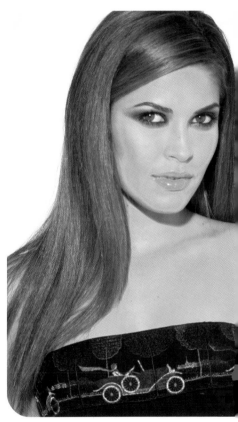

Justine Pasek, Panama, Miss Universe 2002

# the eyes have it

## Porntip "Bui" Nakhirunkanok Simon, Thailand, Miss Universe 1988

Here's something you don't hear from a former beauty queen every day: "I played quarterback for my junior high school football team," says Porntip "Bui" Nakhirunkanok Simon, who grew up in California after leaving her native Thailand at age five. Bui was the kind of girl who built tree houses, shot basketball, and lived on a skateboard.

By the time she entered high school, her outlook began to change. "I became a cheerleader and things just transformed," she recalls. "I was suddenly boy crazy and boys don't like bruises very much." Underneath the sports gear and rough-and-tumble exterior, Bui was a stunning natural beauty. But even as she blossomed headlong into womanhood, her daredevil side remained firmly in place. So when her mother dared Bui to return home to compete for Miss Thailand, she couldn't refuse. "At the time, it was just about the bravest thing I could do," she says. "I figured, if I can get through this, I can get through anything!"

In a time when Thai women still believed it was better to be seen and not heard, Bui's vocal, strong brand of glamour helped her stand out from her rivals on stage. "I was nineteen when I won the Miss Thailand title," she notes. "I was so naive at the time, I wasn't afraid to say anything." The Miss Universe Pageant was set for a mere two weeks after her country's competition—good thing she didn't pass up *that* dare!

Bui has continued to take the world by storm. She's been a tireless crusader for underprivileged children around the world—her Angel's Wings Foundation helped construct homes, boats, and schools in Southeast Asia following the 2004 tsunami.

And did we mention she has a toddler of her own scampering around the house? Suffice it to say, Bui doesn't have much time for extended primping sessions. She wears little to no makeup—she would rather indulge in an occasional facial than bother with foundation. And when it comes to her famously radiant eyes, she swears the sparkle comes from the inside out. "To prevent them from getting puffy and red, I get at least eight hours of sleep, watch alcohol intake, and try to keep stress in check," she says—before admitting to a little outside help. "I love Sisley Double Action Mascara—it not only makes my lashes long, but thick, full, and glamorous."

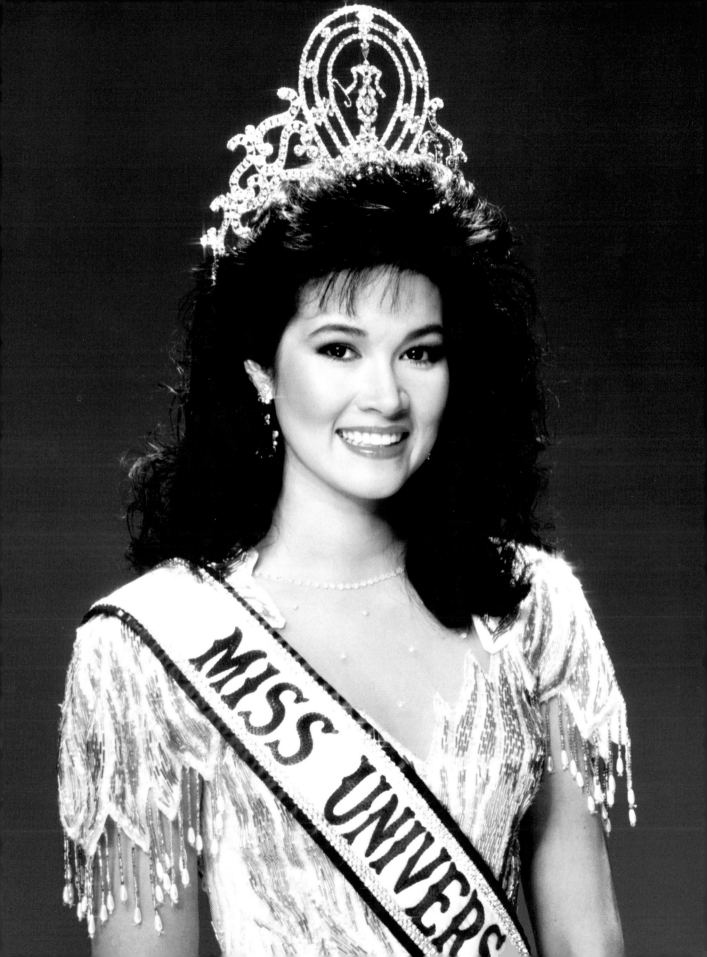

# eye-popping by day

Like Bui Simon, Natalie Glebova (Canada, Miss Universe 2005) firmly believes that eyes really are the windows to the soul. "They're the first thing people notice when they're talking to you, so it's important to play them up to your advantage," she says. "I've always been a big eye makeup person." Natalie switches up her shades and techniques depending on her mood, but her typical daytime look starts with a sheer wash of beige shadow brushed over the lids, all the way up to the brow bone. She applies light brown shadow in the crease. Rather than defining the eyes with conventional liquid liner or pencil, which can look harsh during the day, she smudges a soft line of brown shadow along the upper and lower lashes. After sweeping on a coat of mascara, she glues a few individual lashes at the outer corners to create a subtle, doe-eyed look.

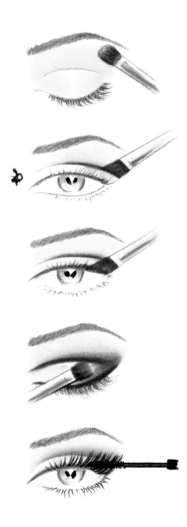

## cheat sheet

CoverGirl makeup artist B.J. Gillian—who regularly works on Miss Universe title-holders and contestants—explains how to create perfect daytime eyes at home.

1. Choose a translucent, slightly shimmery shade that matches your skin. Brush it over the entire lid, from lashes to brow bone.

2. Apply a touch of a deeper, coordinating shade (such as gray, navy, brown, or plum) to the outer portion of the crease for contour.

3. Smudge that deeper shade softly along the upper lash line.

4. Blend both shades together so there are no obvious lines of demarcation, then apply one coat of mascara. (False lashes optional!)

## universal truth

To ensure that eye shadow glides smoothly over the lid, Gillian uses only natural-hair brushes. "I love the CoverGirl Makeup Masters brush because it's the perfect width," he says.

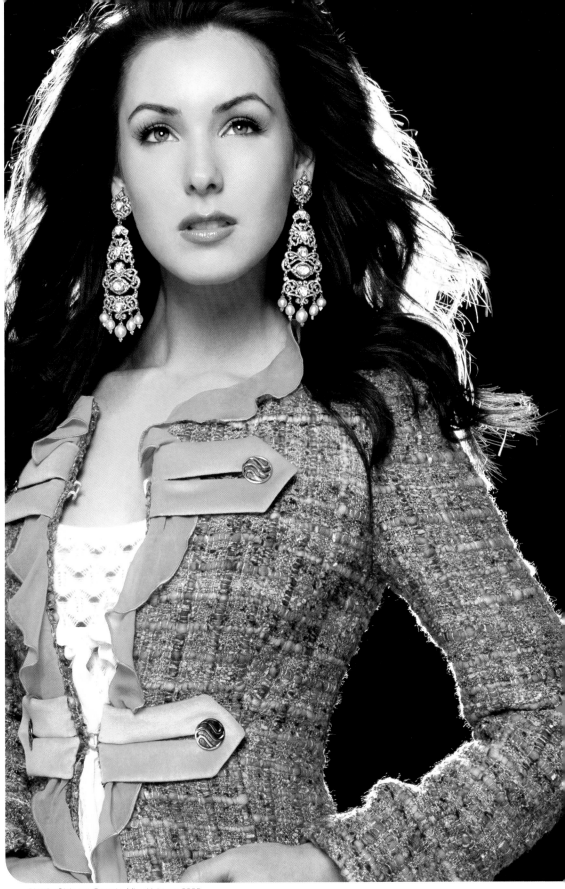

Natalie Glebova, Canada, Miss Universe 2005

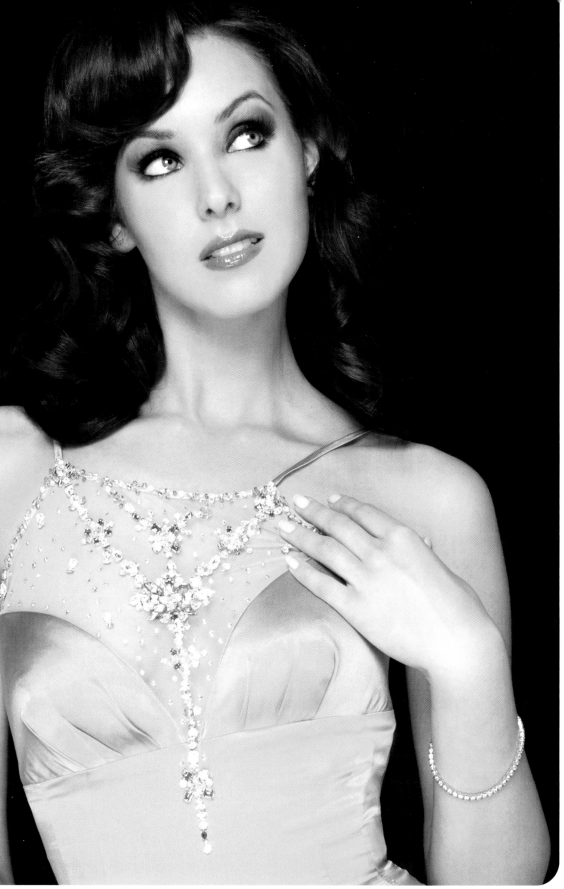

Natalie Glebova, Canada, Miss Universe 2005

# eye-popping by night

Evening eyes are all about drama. As the lights go down and the dress code loosens up, this is your chance to dip into the darker side of the makeup palette and let your sultry side shine through. Natalie Glebova certainly does: After sunset, she keeps the same daytime beige on the lids, then darkens her crease with smoky gray. After adding a touch of shimmery shadow on the brow bone, she applies a full strip of false lashes along the upper lash line.

Applying dark evening eyeliner can be a recipe for disaster if you don't know the proper technique. First, remember that while liquid eyeliner looks more dramatic than pencil and powder, the latter two are easier to control and better bets for the squeamish.

Regardless of which you use, consider this trick from Gillian: Using your nondominant hand, start by gently stretching the outer corner of the lash line, angling it up slightly to separate lashes. Anchor the elbow of your dominant arm on a table, and draw tiny dots of color between individual lashes. In addition to lining the eyes, this makes your fringe appear thicker and more intense. Bonus hint: If using a pencil liner, look for one that comes with a built-in sharpener. The more perfect your point, the better the application.

## cheat sheet

Gillian's secret to amping up the eyes for nighttime: Focus on the crease. Here, he tells us how it's done.

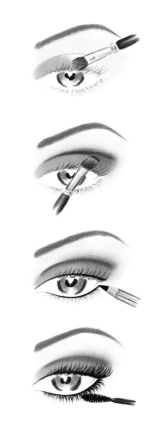

1. Use your favorite shade on the lid, from the lash line to the crease. Feel free to go slightly darker than your daytime color, unless you have very deep-set eyes.

2. Load your brush with a darker shade and press the color into the crease, moving from the outer to the inner corner. Blend the deeper shade so that it extends a bit above and below the crease.

3. Line the upper and lower lash lines with pencil or liquid liner.

4. Curl lashes and apply several coats of mascara.

# luscious lashes

Natalie Glebova (Canada, Miss Universe 2005) knows that spending just a few minutes on your eyelashes can instantly make you look well rested and alert. And if you're a little older than Natalie, a full fringe can even take years off your face. (Just consider how little girls have those enviably long lashes, and you'll know what we mean.) Here, Gillian explains everything you need to know about getting a fabulous fringe.

## curl talk

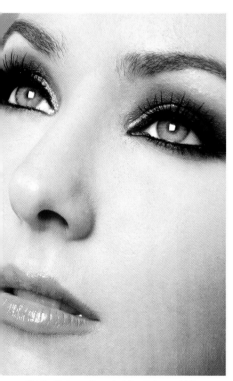

Natalie Glebova, Canada, Miss Universe 2005

The eyelash curler is the most overlooked and underestimated tool of the trade. Once you get the hang of it, it's easy to use—and can make your eyes appear one-third larger. Curling should always be done *before* reaching for the mascara. Here are four steps to gorgeous lashes.

1. Get on your marks. Place your thumb and index finger through the finger tabs of the curler.

2. Get set. Looking down into a mirror, open the curler as far as possible. Slide lashes through the opening of the curler and hold it as close to the base of your lashes as possible.

3. Curl. To curl, bring the thumb and index finger together until the tabs meet. (The idea is to hear them click.) Remember that most curlers take some muscle. If it feels like you're crimping skin, stop and start again.

4. Repeat. Pulse the tabs together gently for twenty seconds, then open. If the curl has an odd bend, move the curler to a different angle and start again.

## universal truth

Wearing a crown hardly makes anyone immune to mascara clumps. To prevent them, make sure the brush itself is free of globs by wiping it with a clean cloth every week or so. Then, after applying mascara, use a metal lash comb to separate lashes.

# the takeaway

Bui Simon avoids waterproof mascaras at all costs because she believes they weaken the lashes. And most experts agree that—unless you're planning on crying or swimming—waterproof just isn't necessary. Those who do use it should invest in an oil-based eye makeup remover, which will dissolve the most durable mascara without scrubbing or tugging, which can harm lashes. Non-waterproof formulas can be rinsed away with an ordinary water-based remover.

## mascara magic

The scores of mascaras lining beauty aisles range in type from waterproof to thickening to lengthening—some actually contain tiny fibers that extend the ends of individual lashes. Choose the one that best suits your needs, in a shade that appeals to you. Rich brown might be a good choice for daytime, while jet black is an ideal evening pick. Here, Gillian explains the ways of the wand.

**Position the wand.** Start by holding the wand horizontally at your lash base.

**Wiggle it, just a little bit.** Use a very subtle side-to-side, zigzag motion from root to tip. This helps ensure that every lash is coated with deep, rich color.

**Go the extra mile.** If you're primping for evening, hold the wand vertically and apply any remaining product on the brush to the bottom lashes in a back and forth motion, like a windshield wiper. Because mascara tends to run when applied to the lower lashes, consider using a clear formula for this area—or leaving the bottom fringe bare.

# the best look for *your* eyes

The Miss Universe Pageant has demonstrated that beautiful eyes come in all sorts of different shapes and sizes—from round to almond-shaped to close-set. This means that eye makeup needs to be just as diverse as the contestants.

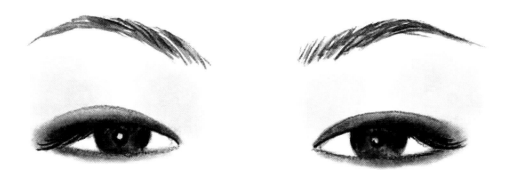

## asian eyes

Bui Simon plays up her top lid by defining it with a pale egg-colored shadow. Then, after locating the indent of her crease with an eye shadow brush, she darkens it slightly with charcoal or dark brown, using that same shade along the lower lash line instead of eyeliner. "With Asian eyes, you can't do anything too dark or heavy, or you'll reduce them to the size of a pea," she says.

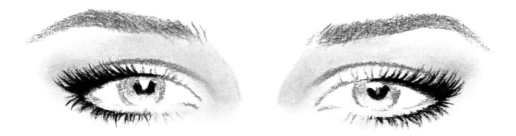

## close-set eyes

Avoid applying eyeliner to the inner corners of the eyes. Instead, start the line at the middle of the pupil and extend, along the top and bottom lash line, emphasizing the outer corners.

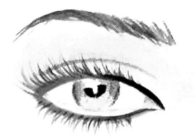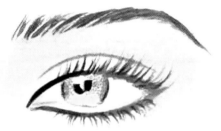

## wide-set eyes

Keep the darkest eyeliner close to the inner corners, then use a liner in a slightly paler shade to define the outer portion of the eyes.

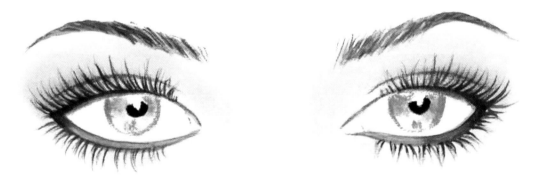

## large eyes

Feel free to apply a bit of liner along the inner rim of the lash line, then smudge it into the lashes.

# unbeatable brows

Grooming the eyebrows is the quickest way to look poised and polished—which is why you'll never catch a reigning Miss Universe with a raggedy, misshapen arch. But just like hemlines and haircuts, pageant-winning brows have evolved over the decades, running the gamut from harsh and overly defined to super-skinny to natural.

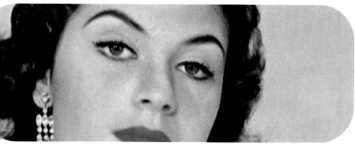

Gladys Zender, Peru, Miss Universe 1957

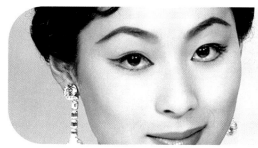

Akiko Kojima, Japan, Miss Universe 1959

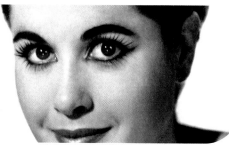

Norma Nolan, Argentina, Miss Universe 1962

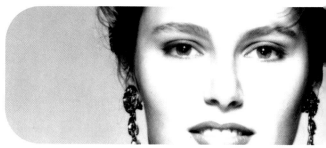

Mona Grudt, Norway, Miss Universe 1990

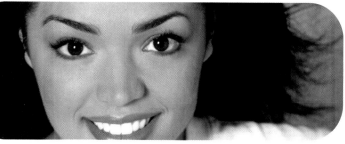

Chelsi Smith, USA, Miss Universe 1995

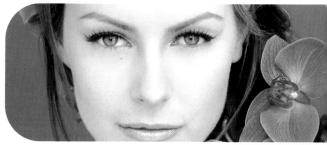

Jennifer Hawkins, Australia, Miss Universe 2004

# do-it-yourself brows

Now the newest (and we think most flattering) standard for brows: naturally full. In other words, women of all cultures are embracing the brows they were born with—cleaning them up just a bit to keep them from looking unkempt or straggly. Miss Universe makeup gurus B.J. Gillian and Linda Rondinella-Osgood guide us through the how-tos.

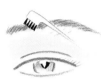

**1. Get the big picture.** To help you see the natural shape of your own eye crease, use a digital camera to snap a picture of the top half of your face with no makeup on.

**2. Brush up.** With a clean brow brush, whisk eyebrows into place—sweeping them up and outward toward the temples.

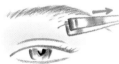

**3. Take some measurements.** Determine the ideal starting and ending points of the brows by holding a pencil flat vertically against your nostril. Observe where the pencil meets the brow area—that should be the start of your brow. Then, angle the pencil so that it aligns with the outer corner of the eye. Wherever it crosses the brow bone is the end point of the brow. It might help to use an eyebrow pencil to mark these points.

**4. Clean up the strays.** Tweeze any stray hairs (above and below) that don't follow the natural shape of your brow and eye crease. Don't forget to pluck hairs between the brows and beyond the end points you've just marked.

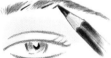

**5. Have your fill.** Fill in bald spots with an eyebrow pencil, using short, light strokes in the direction of hair growth. (Warming the pencil first by rubbing it in the palm of your hand will help it glide more easily.)

**6. Plump 'em up.** Dip a brow brush into a palette of brow powder or eye shadow, then sweep over brows, using quick, feathery strokes. Concentrate most of the powder in the area where hair is thickest.

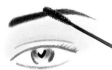

**7. Lock them in place.** Set with brow gel, brushing it up and out toward the arch, then angling brows slightly downward.

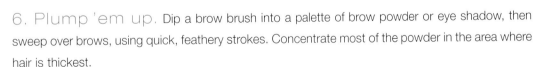

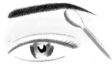

**8. Polish the look.** Clean up any smudges or mistakes with a cotton swab soaked in eye makeup remover.

# tool box

The most beautiful women don't think of going near their eyebrows unless they're armed with the best tools in the world. Here's what your eyebrow "tool box" should include.

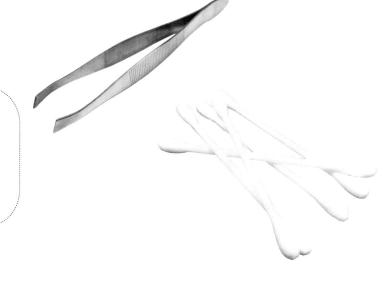

Brushes. The best tool for sweeping arches into place is a spooley, which looks like a large mascara brush. A stiff, angled eyebrow brush is essential for applying brow-filling powder. Many companies sell dual-ended tools containing both brushes.

Gel. Also called brow mascara, this comes in clear or colored. Keeps brows in place with a firm but natural hold.

Pencil. Look for one that doesn't feel too waxy, in a shade that either matches or is slightly lighter than your natural hair color. (However, blondes should choose a shade darker.) Use it to fill holes, not to extend brows.

Powder. Follow the same shade guidelines as for pencil. Use either brow powder or eye shadow to define and extend brows.

Rogaine. Many pros suggest dabbing bald patches with a cotton swab soaked in Rogaine once or twice a day to coax new hair growth. Be sure to keep it away from the eyes.

Tweezers. Choose a pair with a slanted edge—the pointed side will grip the short, stubborn hairs most effectively. Keep tweezers clean and consider having them sharpened (many manufacturers offer this service) every six months to maintain pulling power.

## universal truth

To ensure you have the most flattering eyebrow shape for your face, consider having a professional groom them every six months—then you can maintain them between visits.

# it's all about formula

Eye shadows come in a variety of formulas. Use this guide to find your best fit.

## Pressed powders (in a compact)

*Use it:* If you need durable, long-lasting color, are already wearing loose powder on your lids, or want a formula that's easy to blend and control.

*Lose it:* If you're self-conscious about fine lines. Powder formulas will settle in and exaggerate them.

## Loose powders (in a jar)

*Use it:* If you prefer trendy, slightly shimmery looks, and if you own a good-quality eye shadow brush that you feel very comfortable with.

*Lose it:* If you like the conservative end of the makeup spectrum—or you're a makeup klutz. Unless you're a pro, those shimmery flecks of powder tend to land anywhere but where you want them.

## Creams

*Use it:* If you want a subtler look and are prepared to reapply after a few hours.

*Lose it:* If you want a foolproof formula. Cream shadows are more difficult to manipulate on the skin and take a bit more expertise to pull off.

# do your eyes in seconds

When you're racing to get out the door, cheat your way to prettier peepers by trying one or more of the tricks below.

**Lickety-split liner.** Skip the pencil and liquid. When contouring the crease with eye shadow, smudge that darker color along the lower lashes for instant definition.

**Speedy brow shaper.** When there's no time to truly groom the brows, all you really need is a tinted brow set gel. The brush sweeps arches into place, while the colored goop leaves them looking polished and defined all day.

**Lash fast.** If you can't get to your tube of mascara, rub a bit of oil-free moisturizer between your thumb and index finger and smudge over the lashes. Voilá—they'll look thicker and more lush immediately.

**Stray hair help.** Cover eyebrow stubble with a dab of concealer or creamy eye shadow that matches your skin tone.

**Instant eye-opener.** If you only have time for one thing, make it a curling mascara. Two to three coats lifts, lengthens, and thickens the lashes—and brings the most zombie-like eyes back to the world of the living.

# lip service

## Maritza Sayalero, Venezuela, Miss Universe 1979

Many Miss Universe titleholders say they never much thought about beauty pageants—or beauty in general—until their teen years. Not Maritza Sayalero, the first titleholder from Venezuela. Her mother had once been a runner-up in the Miss Madrid competition. She knew how to take care of herself, and she passed that knowledge on to her daughter.

As a little girl, Maritza would watch her mother carefully applying her makeup, bit by bit. By the time she was fifteen, Maritza was performing the same artistry on her own face—and began blooming before everyone's eyes. "People began to ask me if I would consider entering the Miss Venezuela contest," she remembers. "They said I had the body, the face, and all the things necessary to try it. That was the beginning." Maritza prepared for the local competition for a full year, taking beauty courses, buying styling tools, and playing with her hair color until she found just the right shade. So it's no surprise that she not only ran away with the Miss Venezuela crown, but the Miss Universe crown as well.

Maritza is still deeply committed to most of the beauty lessons she learned years ago. She keeps her hair strong and healthy with deep conditioning treatments, and she's an expert at contouring her cheekbones. And her highest-ranking glamour essential fits easily into the front pocket of her purse: lipstick. "I love lipstick—I can't go outside without it," she says. "I don't care if I don't have blush or foundation on. But I always have to have lipstick. It gives my face more color and makes it look healthy."

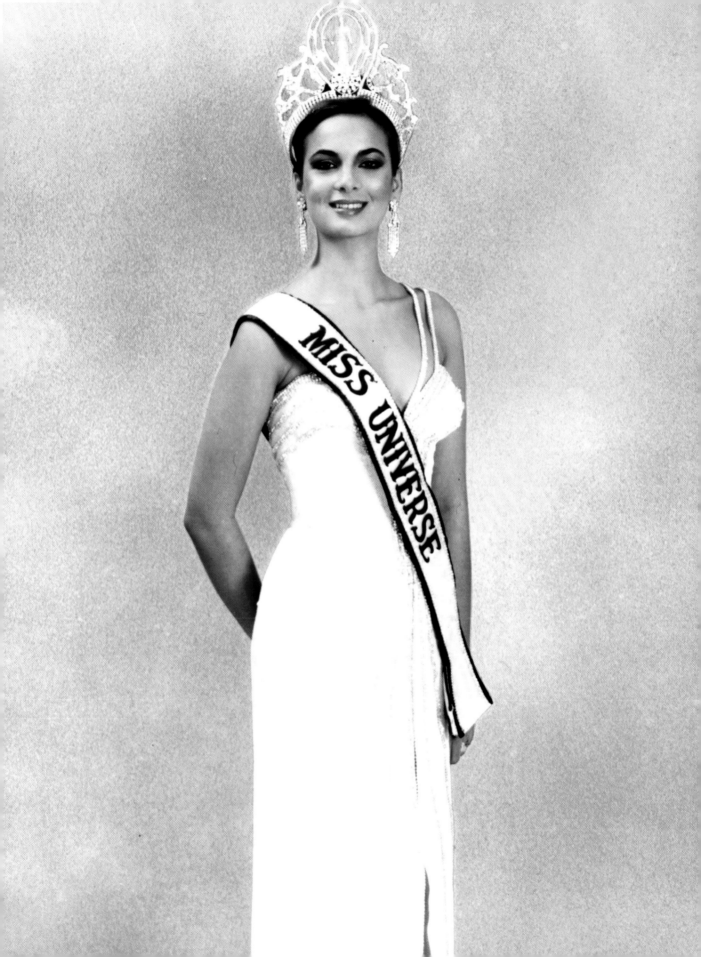

# finding your perfect pucker

If the right lip color can make the entire face look brighter, clearer, and more radiant, the wrong one can make an otherwise great complexion look deathly. According to CoverGirl's B.J. Gillian, a Miss Universe makeup artist, a quick way to determine your approximate shade range is to peek in your jewelry box. "If you love silver, chances are you have cool-based undertones and should choose lip color with silvery-blue undertones," he says. "If you feel good in gold, you likely have warm-based undertones and should select shades that have yellow-golden undertones.

Still not sure? Whether you prefer a soft palette or a more dramatic one, take a cue from these crown winners.

## the soft side

Fair skin is best flattered by pale pinks and berries.

Medium and olive skin looks pretty with apricots, beiges, and bronzy nudes.

Dark skin is complemented by mauves, sheer reds, and berries.

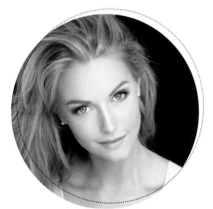

Jennifer Hawkins
Australia, Miss Universe 2004

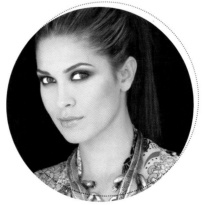

Justine Pasek
Panama, Miss Universe 2002

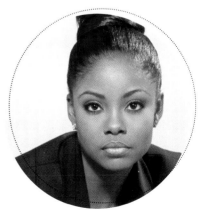

Wendy Fitzwilliam
Trinidad & Tobago, Miss Universe 1998

# balancing act

To wear deep, dramatic lip color without looking clownish, play down the rest of the face with a soft shade of blush and minimal eye makeup.

A pale, sheer mouth won't look washed out if you pair it with intense smoky eye makeup and well-defined brows.

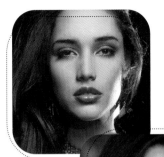

Amelia Vega
Dominican Republic
Miss Universe 2003

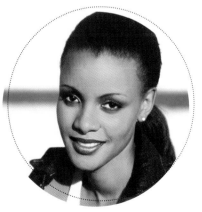

## the sultry side

**Fair skin** looks warm and inviting with deep berries and rich wines.

**Medium and olive skin** glows when accented by brown and raisin tones.

**Dark skin** gets gorgeous with burgundies and plums.

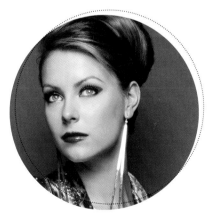

Jennifer Hawkins
Australia, Miss Universe 2004

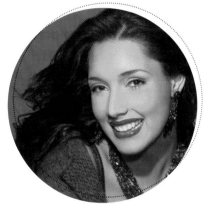

Amelia Vega
Dominican Republic, Miss Universe 2003

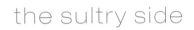

Mpule Kwelagobe
Botswana, Miss Universe 1999

# apply yourself

To give the mouth extra staying power during the Miss Universe Pageant, makeup artists load on the liner, lipstick, and loose powder before sending contestants to the stage. Maximizing your pout's longevity for real life isn't all that different. Here's how to pucker like you mean it.

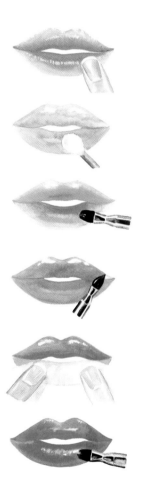

**1. Begin with a balm.** Hydrate the lips with a nongreasy balm. Avoid anything too slick, as anything you apply on top will slip right off. Wait ten to fifteen minutes for the balm to be absorbed into the lips.

**2. Clean the surface.** Remove excess balm and flakes by sweeping a cotton swab across the lips.

**3. Colorize your mouth.** With a lip brush, paint the center of the mouth using short strokes, gradually blending it outward. Stop just before you reach the corners. Start with a thin layer of lipstick, and add one more if you need it.

**4. Line up.** Many experts feel that lip pencils tend to look harsh and severe. A more modern approach to defining the lips: After applying lipstick, outline your mouth with the tip of your brush. If you're worried about color bleeding into fine lines, apply an anti-feathering product just outside the lips' borders.

**5. Take a powder.** Hold one ply of tissue to your mouth, and gently pat over the tissue once with loose powder (just enough powder will sift through the tissue). Reapply one thin layer of lipstick, then dot the center of the lips with clear gloss.

## universal truth

Natalie Glebova (Canada, Miss Universe 2005) says that her mouth's borders aren't naturally defined, so she feels that lip pencil is a must. "But I don't like the look of harshly lined lips," she says. Her beautiful compromise: a neutral lip liner that matches the color of her mouth—and leaves no telltale ring when lipstick starts to fade. Many companies make clear gel liners that serve this same purpose.

Angela Visser (Holland, Miss Universe 1989) has kept the same color of lipstick in her purse for years. "It's not a bright pink or a dark purple, but somewhere in between," she says. "I've always worn it." More often than not, however, Angela prefers the natural look of tinted lip balm. She adores Body Shop's Born Lippy Strawberry because "it looks really lush and glossy, and it feels so nice going on." Angela isn't alone: Glosses and balms offer a fresh, subtle way to dress up the mouth—with minimal labor. Here's how to maximize their potential.

### Choose the right formula.
Lose the super-shiny, sticky formulas. Those old-school glosses will make you look like a teenybopper—or worse, as if you're drooling. Pick ones that glide on without feeling tacky and contain barely perceptible shimmer particles instead of hard-core frost.

### Use a light hand.
"The key to wearing lip gloss is to remember that less is more," says B.J. Gillian. "Apply only to the bottom lip and press lips together to assure you get just the right amount of gloss for your mouth."

### Take it with you.
The bad news about glosses and balms is that they don't have a ton of staying power. The good news: Smudges are hardly noticeable, so you can apply—and reapply—them anywhere with your finger. No mirror required.

### Dress in layers.
Can't bear to give up your full-bodied lipstick but still want the dewy look of gloss? Simply top your favorite lipstick with a thin coat of gloss or balm. In fact, a dot of shine in the center of your lips will make thin lips appear fuller.

### Act your age.
If you have a lot of wrinkling around your mouth, consider skipping gloss altogether. Anything remotely shiny magnifies fine lines. A matte lip balm, however, is still fine and can be a good way to plump up a pout that has lost moisture with age.

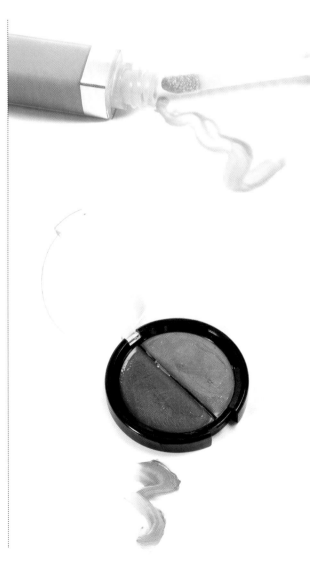

# tool box

Those who opt for a mere touch of gloss on the mouth don't need more than an index finger. But anyone who's more serious about her lipstick requires a bit more in the way of supplies.

Lip brush. Palette lipsticks usually come with a lip brush, but having a spare comes in handy if you want to brush on a formula that comes in a tube or pot. The best brushes have short, stiff bristles for a precise application.

Lip color. Once you've found your ideal lip shade family, it's a good idea to buy it in a few different consistencies. For example, if you like berries, consider looking for a berry-toned lipstick that's creamy and opaque, another that's a bit more sheer, and a super-light gloss or balm.

Lip liner. Lip liner certainly is not required, but if you feel your lips need extra definition, choose a liner that either matches your lips or glides on sheer.

Makeup remover. This is absolutely essential if your favorite lipsticks are even remotely heavy. A good, oil-based formula will dissolve any pigment instantly—without harsh rubbing and scrubbing. Applied with a cotton swab, it's also useful for cleaning up post-application smudges around the lips.

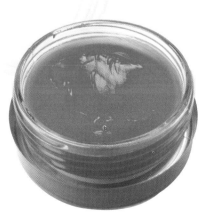

Keeping your lips looking lovely is tricky business—unless you have a good cheat sheet to work from. Try these tips.

Lock it in place. If you don't have an anti-feathering formula handy, apply a touch of translucent loose powder just outside the mouth's borders with a clean eye shadow brush before putting on lipstick. This will keep color from sneaking into fine lines.

Get rich quick. Who says only gloss and balms can be applied with your fingers? If you want the drama of a dark lipstick—but don't have time to reach for a mirror and brush—dab it on the center of the mouth with your index finger and press lips together. The result: a slightly stained mouth without the sculpted look usually associated with rich lipstick.

Fatten up. For those with thin lips, extending your lipstick a hair beyond the pucker's natural border is allowed—but do so only at the Cupid's bow in the center. Trying to fake a full lip near the edges of the mouth can easily look clownish.

Protect your pearly whites. Any pageant winner worth her crown knows how to keep lipstick from staining the teeth: Wrap your lips around your finger as if you're sucking on it, then slowly slide it out to remove color on your inner lips.

Take good care. Treat your lips well and they'll look beautiful even when bare. That means wearing a balm containing SPF during any prolonged sun exposure and slicking on a super-hydrating lip moisturizer just before bed. Occasional gentle exfoliation with a soft toothbrush will also help keep the lips soft and smooth.

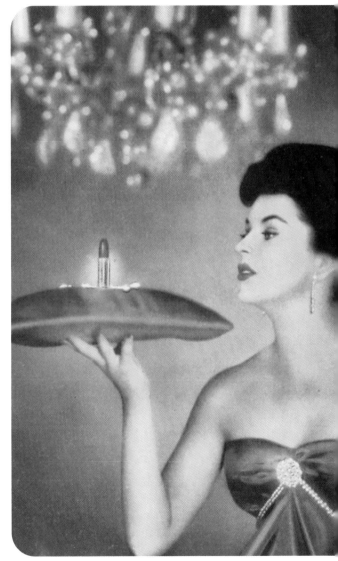

Luz Marina Zuluaga, Colombia, Miss Universe 1958

# CHAPTER 8

# nailing it

## Margaret Gardiner, South Africa, Miss Universe 1978

Anyone who doubts that Miss Universe contestants truly get along like sisters should talk to Margaret Gardiner. "We had a great group of girls," says the South African native—who wound up sharing a New York City apartment with her first runner-up for five years after her win. "And Miss England was hilarious," she recalls. "I swear I won the contest because of her. While we sat on the stage, she gave a running dialogue of what was going on with very funny observations. I was laughing so hard, but to the audience it looked like I was simply smiling."

Beneath the smiles, Margaret was struggling to answer questions, from journalists and judges alike, about the turbulent political and racial climate in her country. She admits now that she had a tough time coping with her sudden fame—which is partly why she ducked out of the spotlight at the end of her reign to earn a degree in psychology. Margaret eventually returned to the cameras, first to cohost a morning television program in South Africa, and more recently, to interview A-list celebrities for an entertainment show.

Clearly, Margaret was never the type to claw her way to the top—which is a good thing, because she doesn't have the nails for it. Keeping her nails healthy and filed short is her usual MO. "I'd rather shoot hoops with my son," she says. "I think it's tacky to have very, very long nails. Surprisingly, many of the actresses I interview have short nails without colored polish. But if I'm going to an event, I'll take the time to do a home manicure."

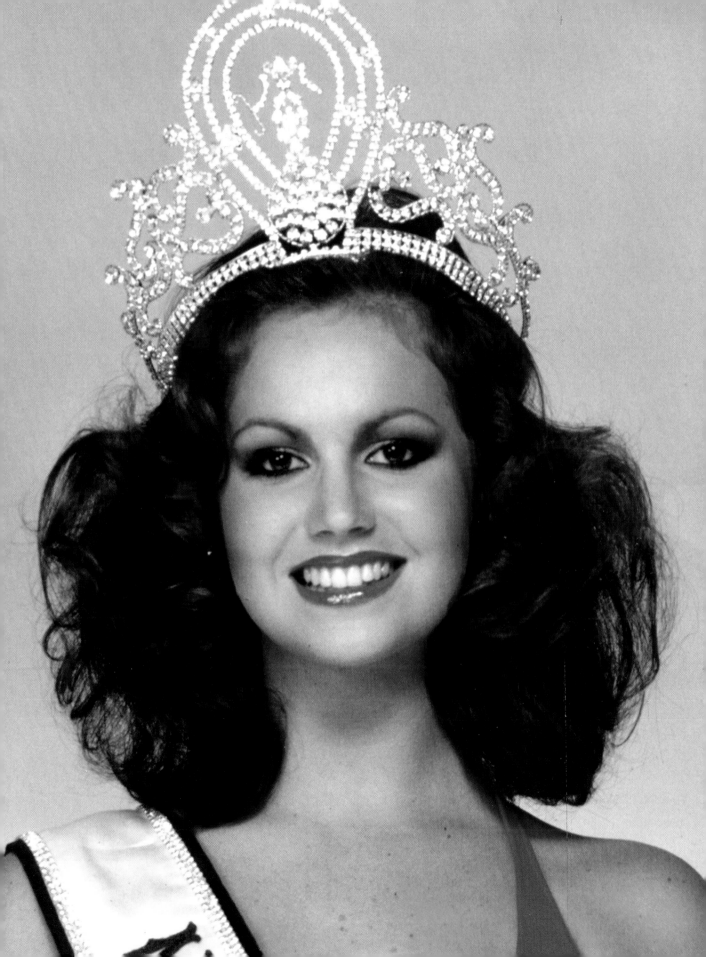

# the universal manicure

Giving yourself a manicure not only saves time and money—it's also a great way to unwind after a hectic day. After all, this is one of the few times you're actually *forced* to sit still. The biggest trick to attaining flawless, chip-free results is to give yourself loads of time. Wait until your favorite television show is on, and take care of any hand-related tasks (doing dishes, paying bills) before you sit down with your polish. You want to allow your nails to dry for an hour, if at all possible. Here's how to proceed.

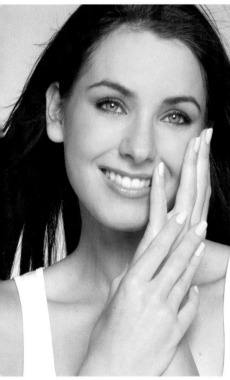

Natalie Glebova, Canada, Miss Universe 2005

1. Clean up. Using a cotton ball soaked in nonacetone remover (it's less drying than conventional formulas), wipe away all traces of existing polish.

2. Find your shape. With a fine-grade nail file, file the nails in one direction to the desired length and shape—rounded squares are not only flattering, but prevent weak nails from breaking.

3. Buff them down. Use a soft buffer to smooth the surface of each nail. But don't overdo it, or you'll risk weakening your nails.

4. Help your hands. Soak your fingers in a bowl of warm, soapy water for five minutes, then use a hand or body scrub to exfoliate your hands. Rinse, then slather your hands with moisturizing cream.

5. Tidy your talons. Brush cuticle oil on the base of each nail. Use an orangewood stick to gently push back the cuticles (don't cut them), then wrap cotton around the stick, dip it in polish remover, and whisk it over the nails to dissolve surface oils that can keep polish from adhering.

6. Smooth out the rough spots. Brush on a ridge-filling base coat, and let it dry for two minutes.

7. Finger paint. Apply one thin coat of your favorite polish, wait three minutes, then apply a second thin coat. Make sure to polish the very tips—and even the underside of the nail—to prevent premature chipping.

8. Top it off. Brush on a clear top coat, and let the nails dry for at least twenty minutes—but two hours is best. (Quick-dry top coats, while convenient, are more prone to chipping.)

9. Mend your mistakes. Dip a sponge-tip eye-shadow applicator or a cotton-wrapped orangewood stick in polish remover, and carefully clean up smudged skin.

# universal truth ♕

It's been said before, but it certainly bears repeating: Like so many of her fellow Miss Universe veterans, Margaret Gardiner swears her best secret for keeping hands youthful and soft is sunscreen. "You can get fried driving your car," she says. "I've taken to wearing hand protection. And I try to drive with gloves on."

## application perfection

No doubt, the hardest part of do-it-yourself nails is applying the polish. Here's one hint: When painting with your nondominant hand, maximize your control by resting it on a book an inch or two above the table. And whether you're working on your hands or your feet, use this polishing technique to achieve the most flawless application.

1. Pare down the polish. While removing the wand from the bottle, press the brush against the bottle's lip to squeeze out excess fluid. This will ensure the thinnest possible coat. (Heavy coats are more likely to bubble and chip.)

2. Find your position. Place the tip of the brush an eighth of an inch above the nail base. Let the bristles fan out.

3. Work in threes. Paint a thin layer of polish down the middle, then on each side. You should only need three strokes to paint each nail—fewer if working on small toenails.

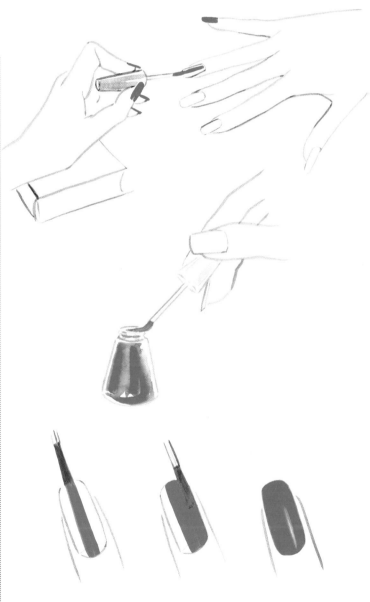

# universal truth

Swab the surface of yellowed or stained nails with hydrogen peroxide (no more than once a month) to brighten them. Or add a teaspoon of peroxide to your soaking water.

# the universal pedicure

The notion of tending to your toes may seem a tad unappealing, but executing a home pedicure is actually an easy way to turn your bathroom into a four-star luxury spa. Margaret Gardiner incorporates her foot treatments into an overall body soak in her Jacuzzi. "If any rough patches appear, I attack them with a pumice, then lavish cream on them as many times a day as time will allow," she says.

1. **Dispense with the old.** Soak a cotton ball in nonacetone remover and strip away existing polish.

2. **Cut them short.** Clip the nails straight across (this will prevent ingrowns) so that they're level or just below the tips of the toes. Then round the corners slightly with a nail file.

3. **Find a buffer zone.** Use a soft buffing block to smooth ridges on the nail surfaces—but remember that overbuffing can thin and weaken nails.

4. **Treat your tootsies.** Soak your feet in a tub of warm, soapy water for at least five minutes—for an extra treat, add a few drops of lavender or lemon oil.

5. **Don't be so callous.** Rub your feet with a grainy scrub. Slough away dead skin on thickened spots like the heels and soles with a damp loofah or pumice.

6. **Get mega-moisture.** Rinse away all traces of soap and scrub, then massage in a rich foot or body cream.

7. **Make your toes glow.** Pat your feet dry with a fluffy towel, then rub cuticle oil into the base of each nail. Push back the cuticles with an orangewood stick (don't cut them). Then wind cotton around the stick, dip it in polish remover, and clean the nail surfaces.

8. **Remove the ridges.** Apply a ridge-filling base coat and wait two minutes.

9. **Just add color.** Brush on two thin coats of polish, followed by a clear top coat, waiting three minutes between each.

10. **Make it perfect.** Soak an orangewood stick wrapped in cotton or a clean eye shadow applicator in polish remover to remove smudges and mistakes around the nails.

● ● ● ● ● ●

## in her own words

"I think having a good pedicure—whether at home or in a salon—is one of the most important things a woman can do for herself. If you've gone to the trouble of buying gorgeous shoes before going to meet a guy for coffee, the last thing you want him to do is look down and see raggedy cuticles all over the place. I've always tried to do the pedicure thing every two weeks—at least."

—Jennifer Hawkins,
Australia, Miss Universe 2004

# made in the shade

Jennifer Hawkins happily tended her own nails until she won the crown in 2004. And for that year, it was salons and spas appointments galore. Jennifer briefly embraced French manicures, but soon found how difficult they were to maintain. "Now I stick with clear pink on my hands," she says, "and watermelons and pinks on my toes." Most women tend to wear more neutral shades on their fingers, saving the brighter ones for the feet, but the more important rule of thumb is to use a color palette that flatters your skin tone.

## the pales

Fair skin: Try cool, blue-based pale pinks and light berries. Avoid lavender or yellow-based shades.

Medium and olive skin: Try white-pinks and gold-flecked sheers. Avoid anything with a bluish undertone.

Dark skin: Try bright pinks or beige- and yellow-toned sheers. Avoid shades that look very chalky on the nails.

## the darks

Fair skin: Try cool, deep berries, blood red, and plum. Avoid browns and bright purples.

Medium and olive skin: Try rusty brown, orange-based red, and deep maroon. Avoid berries.

Dark skin: Try rich brown, cream, and deep plum. Avoid nothing—dark skin looks good with just about anything.

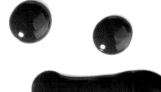

Maybe one reason Margaret Gardiner doesn't spend much time prettying her nails is that she treats them like gold. "When I'm looking for something in my purse, I use a pen to scoot things around so my nails don't get chipped or torn," she says. She slides that same pen beneath CD and DVD wrappers, rather than using her nails to peel them open. Here's how to keep your manicure going long past its expiration date.

**Let it dry.** Polish can remain tacky and easily dented an hour after it's applied. If you can possibly spend a full hour doing nothing with your hands (or toes), you'll be rewarded with a week's worth of smooth, shiny nails.

**Wear gloves.** Gardening and washing dishes can be murder on nails. A pair of latex mitts will protect them from water, harsh cleaners, and other hazardous materials.

**Invest in nail insurance.** Reapply your clear top coat every other day to prevent chipping at the tips.

**Save your skin.** Keep a loofah and pumice stone in the shower, so that you can slough away calluses before they get out of hand.

**Moisturize, moisturize, moisturize!** To keep your hands, feet, and cuticles hydrated, reapply a rich cream several times a day. Before bed, slip on a pair of cotton socks over freshly moisturized feet—they'll feel baby-soft by morning.

## universal truth

Barbara Palacios (Venezuela, Miss Universe 1986) has a secret weapon for keeping her nails shiny and beautifully strong: olive oil. "I rub it into my nails after I wash dishes or do anything that's harsh on my hands," she says.

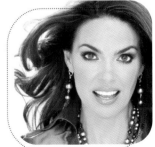

Barbara Palacios, Venezuela
Miss Universe 1986

# the tool box

To keep their nails looking presentable between manicure and pedicure appointments, titleholders arm themselves with soap, files, and gentle polish removers. Here are the essentials that will keep your feet and hands happy.

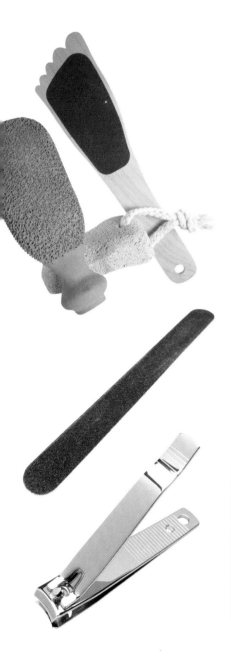

Buffer. The best have two sides—a textured one to reduce bumps and a super-soft one to shine and remove stains.

Clippers. The sharper they are, the cleaner the cut, so it's worth the extra money to invest in a good-quality pair. And because all clippers dull over time, replace them at least every two years.

Cuticle oil. Good ones contain essential oils, such as grapeseed oil, to nourish parched cuticles. Most pros advise against snipping away the skin, so skip the cuticle remover.

Nail file. Fine-grade versions shape nails without tearing or breaking them. Fiberglass files—Diamoncel makes a great one—last far longer than the disposable kind, provided you clean them periodically with soap and water.

Orangewood stick. From chipping away grime to pushing back cuticles to cleaning away smudges—the uses for these unassuming tools go on and on.

Remover. To dissolve polish without overdrying the nails, choose a remover without acetone. Some formulas even contain aloe to help restore moisture.

Ridge filler. This doubles as a base coat, smoothing out uneven nail beds and preventing colored polish from staining your talons.

Scrubbers. Keep a grainy body exfoliating cleanser, along with a loofah and a pumice stone, in your bathroom to keep calluses from getting out of hand.

Toe separators. These prevent your toes from getting too cozy during and after your pedicure, while your nails are drying.

Top coat. Don't think about skimping on it. The top coat provides more than just shine—it can double the longevity of your manicure.

# how to do your nails in no time

Whether you're a reigning beauty queen or a mother of four, sitting still long enough to polish your nails (then let them dry) isn't always realistic. Fortunately, there are speedier ways to make your hands and feet look presentable.

Bag it. For a no-scrub way to smooth away rough spots, fill two plastic bags with rich body cream or foot cream, pop them in the microwave for fifteen to thirty seconds (be sure they're warm, not hot), then immerse your hands or feet in the goop. Wait five minutes, then massage in any cream left on the skin.

Buff your way beautiful. A good buffing will impart a natural shine that looks almost as good as a coat of clear nail polish. The bonus, notes Margaret Gardiner, is that giving nails a week or two off between polishes "lets them breathe and maintains their healthy color."

Resort to quickie polishes. While quick-dry polishes and top coats aren't nearly as durable as conventional ones, they're fine to use in a pinch. Just be doubly sure to reapply your top coat every other day to preserve the job as long as possible.

Grow longer nails in minutes. To add the illusion of length without resorting to falsies (which can damage nail beds), paint one thick column of neutral-colored polish up the center of the nail, leaving a very thin strip of bare nail on either side.

Fix a chip. The quickest way to make chipped polish look as good as new: Start by gently buffing the spot until it feels smooth to the touch. Fill it with the same polish you're wearing, wait three minutes, then paint the entire nail with polish. Finish with a quick-dry top coat.

# the smile that beguiles

## Angela Visser, Holland, Miss Universe 1989

Angela Visser is a natural beauty in the truest sense of the word. She grew up in a small village outside Rotterdam, Holland, surrounded by rolling green fields. "I always remember being outside," she says. "People there were always gardening, walking, and playing tennis and golf. I spent a lot of time on my bicycle, and when you're on a bicycle, you can't really wear high heels."

Not that Angela was a tomboy. She idolized Brigitte Bardot as a teenager (and still does!) and read her share of fashion magazines. But it wasn't until friends encouraged her to enter the Miss Holland contest that she had a chance to immerse herself in all things girly. She won easily, continued to the Miss Universe contest—and immediately worried that she was in way over her head. "I remember arriving and seeing a lot of women with a lot of suitcases," she says.

In the end, the girl without all the excess baggage ran away with the crown. Angela parlayed her Miss Universe victory into a successful acting and modeling career before shifting gears in 2005 to focus on her latest (and most special) project—raising her daughter, Amelie.

It's no wonder the Dutch beauty sails through life with a glowing smile. Angela—who has never whitened her teeth—suspects that her wholesome upbringing is the main factor behind her megawatt mouth. "Everything we ate over there was fresh," she says. "Lots of fruits and vegetables. And I drank milk—pretty much straight from the cow—like kids in America drink soda. But I'm sure good genes have something to do with it, too."

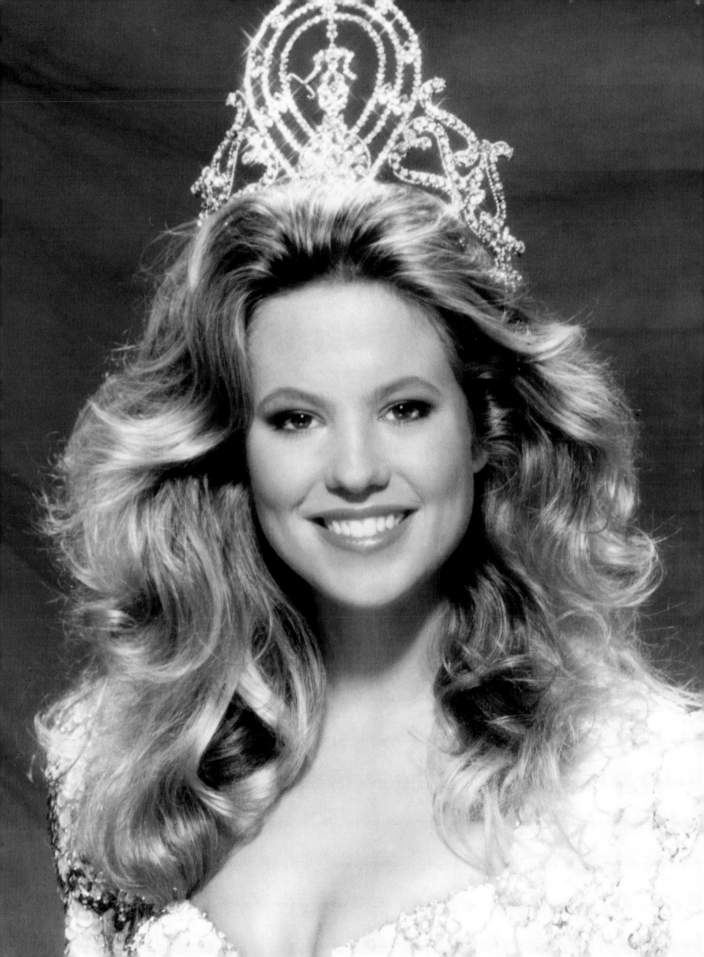

# look on the bright side

Angela Visser says that she never smoked a cigarette or sipped red wine in her life, and that she rarely drinks coffee. Take one look at her smile and you know she's telling the truth. Stains are caused by a variety of factors, most often from particles that are deposited on the teeth while eating or drinking. Diet is one factor that determines how easily your teeth will discolor, but the thickness and composition of your teeth are also key. So is age—the older you are, the more stubborn stains tend to be.

## the causes of stains

There are four basic types of discoloration. Surface stains, caused by smoking and coffee drinking, develop on tooth enamel and usually respond well to whitening treatments. Age-related stains strike the inner portion of the tooth— yellow ones can often be bleached, while grayish stains are more resistant. Intrinsic stains (usually caused by child- hood antibiotic use, flouride treatments, or prolonged high fever) tend to be black, brown, or gray, and typically don't improve much with bleaching treatments. Finally, stains caused by a trauma to the tooth (think root canal) appear as a gray or brown cast. Bleach will help some of these discolorations, but not all.

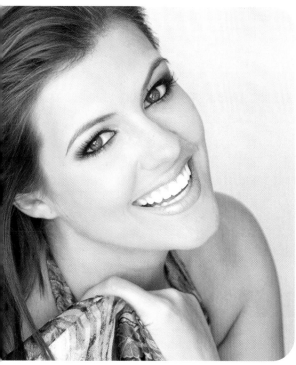

Chelsea Cooley, Miss USA 2005

## lighten up

New York City dentist Radford Y. Goto has whitened the teeth of every sitting Miss Universe (not to mention Miss USA and Miss Teen USA) since 2000. He has a secret whitening weapon: a system called BriteSmile. The treatment bleaches teeth in just over an hour, using a special lamp to speed-activate the hydrogen peroxide spread over the teeth. For those who prefer not to spend time and money in the doctor's office, at-home treatments offer a more economical alternative. They can be effective on mild, superficial stains, and most dentists don't see much wrong with trying them. (Though they say it is always best to see a professional to make sure that discoloration isn't due to something more serious, like a cavity or infection.) One caveat: Whitening products, whether sold by a doctor or a drugstore, deliver purely cosmetic benefits—they should never be substi- tuted for a dental cleaning and checkup.

# from the drugstore

**Toothpastes and gels:** While any old toothpaste will help clean away surface grime and discoloration, whitening formulas contain additional ingredients and abrasives to break down more stubborn stains, but most don't contain peroxide. They can definitely give your smile that extra polish, but don't expect the dramatic results of a bleaching treatment.

*The risks:* Little to none—though you may experience slightly increased tooth sensitivity. Also, to be sure the formula is cleansing properly, check the package for the American Dental Association seal of approval.

**Paint-ons:** Brush these over the teeth either during the day or at night, depending on the formula. The peroxide gel clings to the surface, bleaching stains on (and just below) the outer enamel.

*The risks:* Virtually none, except possible mild tooth sensitivity. But because your saliva may dilute the gel, it may not work as well as products that seal bleach against the teeth with a barrier.

**Strips:** Thin plastic strips coated with peroxide gel wrap around top and lower teeth, forming a barrier to prevent saliva from diluting the bleach ingredients.

*The risks:* Possible mild tooth sensitivity. Also, keep in mind that strips usually don't reach the back teeth, so expect those to remain yellowed.

**Trays:** Plastic trays filled with peroxide gel hold the bleach firmly against teeth and between spaces. Depending on the brand and type, some trays are worn overnight, while others can be used for an hour during the day. Most come in one standard size, but a few can be molded to the shape of your mouth after a soak in hot water.

*The risks:* Because this method delivers the most concentrated dose of bleach, sensitivity is much more common. Another unwanted side effect: red, irritated, sometimes lightened gums. This will go away once treatment is discontinued.

# from the dentist

**Take-home trays:** These dentist-prescribed trays work better than the drugstore variety for two reasons: First, they contain a higher concentration of bleach (usually over 20 percent peroxide compared to levels of 9 percent or less for over-the-counter trays). Second, trays are precisely molded to fit your mouth, which ensures that gel stays firmly against the teeth—and doesn't migrate to the gum area. Most patients wear them for several weeks, either overnight or for thirty minutes a day.

*The risks:* Again, the most common complaint is tooth sensitivity. But because this is done under a dentist's supervision, your dentist can monitor the fit and gel concentration to make you more comfortable.

**Power bleaching:** Treatments such as Zoom and BriteSmile are ideal for those without a lot of time or patience. After a peroxide gel is brushed over the teeth, a light or laser is focused over the teeth to help bleach penetrate quickly. Expect to be in the chair for three twenty-minute cycles, but most dentists have DVD players and other forms of entertainment to fight boredom.

*The risks:* Nothing that hasn't been said before. However some experts think that, unless you have a wedding or an event coming up in the next week, you're better off with dentist-prescribed trays, which tend to give more thorough, long-lasting results. (Many dentists send patients home with trays after power-bleaching teeth.)

# miles of smiles

Whitening, bonding, and veneers may be a relatively recent phenomenon, but gorgeous grins have always been in style. Here's a look back on some of Miss Universe's most dazzling smiles.

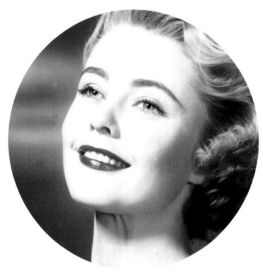

Hellevi Rombin, Sweden, Miss Universe 1955

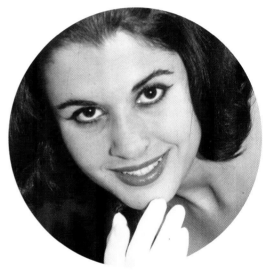

Norma Nolan, Argentina, Miss Universe 1962

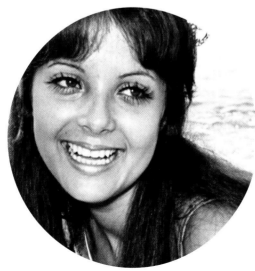

Marisol Malaret, Puerto Rico, Miss Universe 1970

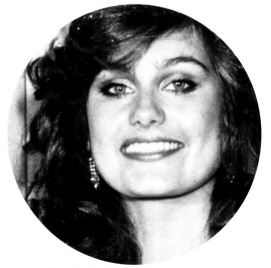

Karen Baldwin, Canada, Miss Universe 1982

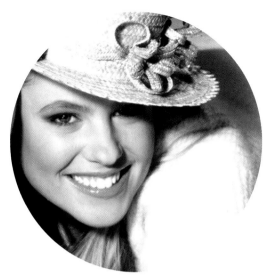
Angela Visser, Holland, Miss Universe 1989

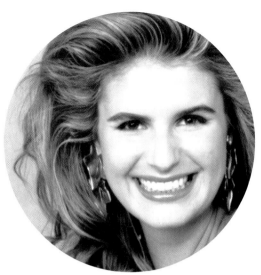
Michelle McLean, Namibia, Miss Universe 1992

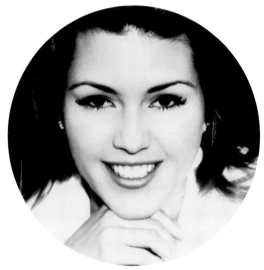
Alicia Machado, Venezuela, Miss Universe 1996

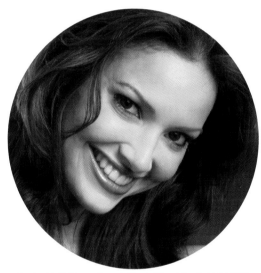
Denise M. Quiñones August, Puerto Rico, Miss Universe 2001

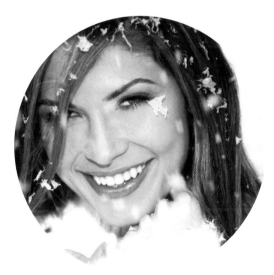
Justine Pasek, Panama, Miss Universe 2002

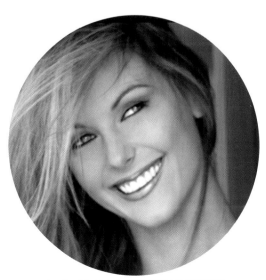
Jennifer Hawkins, Australia, Miss Universe 2004

# say cheese!

Bleaching is only one option on cosmetic dentistry's ever-expanding menu. Which means even women with crooked, chipped, or missing teeth can pay their way to a pageant-perfect smile. (And we do mean *pay*—these treatments don't come cheap.) Cosmetic dentist Allyson K. Hurley explains some of the most popular procedures she performs.

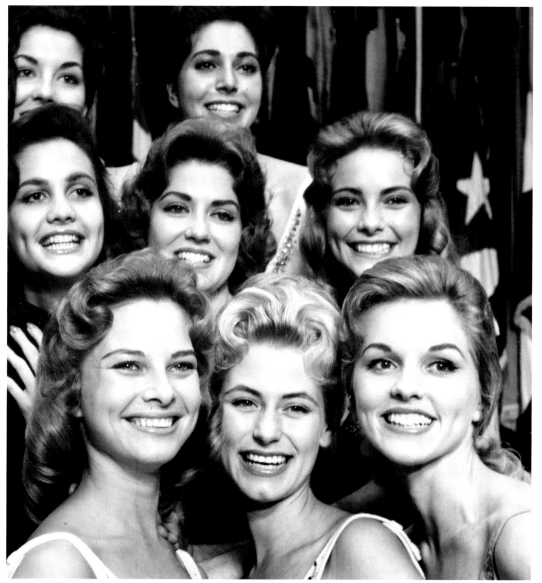

Miss Universe contestants,1960

Braces: Don't turn the page yet—braces have come a long way since the railroad versions everyone endured in seventh grade. Today's clear braces shift teeth into place with invisible wires attached to porcelain brackets. And if your smile isn't severely crooked, you may be able to get away with a device called Invisalign—a set of clear, removable plastic aligners that slowly straighten teeth.

*The cost*: Several thousand dollars, depending on type and amount of time braces stay on.

*Keep in mind:* Clear braces cost significantly more than old-school metal versions. And regardless of which straightening method you use, results can take months or even years to fully materialize.

Bonding: A white composite material is applied to correct chips, fill gaps, mend cracks, and change the shape of a tooth. Once the material is molded around the tooth, it's hardened with a light source, then polished until it matches the rest of your teeth.

*The cost:* $400–$1,000 per tooth.

*Keep in mind:* While bonding has a much lower per-tooth cost than veneers (see below), results don't last nearly as long. Expect bonding to last about five years. Also remember that the bonding material stains more easily than veneers.

Veneers: Unlike crowns, which fit around an entire tooth, veneers are custom-made porcelain shells that are bonded to the tooth exterior. To help veneers attach properly, the dentist files down your original tooth (the uneven surface increases adhesion). Whether they're fitted over several teeth at a time or just one, veneers can change the shape of your smile, cover a chip or crack, or camouflage discoloration that's resistant to bleaching.

*The cost:* $1,100–$2,000 per tooth.

*Keep in mind:* Veneers generally last anywhere from five to fifteen years. That means you'll almost certainly have to pony up for another at least once in your lifetime—because you can't simply go back to your old teeth once those porcelain laminates wear out.

Gum lifting: If you're self-conscious about your "gummy" grin, this procedure can help. The dentist uses a laser to remove excess gum tissue and reshape the gums—with minimal pain and often no blood. Results last forever.

*The cost:* $500 per tooth.

*Keep in mind:* You want to choose a cosmetic dentist who really knows her way around a laser device to lessen the risk of complications.

# tool box

Between dental visits, you need more than bleaching trays to keep your smile shiny, clean, and healthy. Is your bathroom properly stocked?

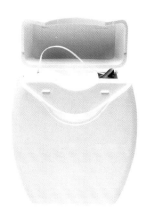

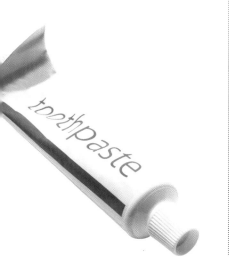

Bleach. You can choose from a wealth of types and brands of bleaches. But consider seeing your dentist before starting any whitening program.

Chewing gum. You read right. Chomping on a piece of sugarless gum between meals increases saliva flow, which helps wash away food particles and decay-causing acids.

Dental floss. Floss comes waxed, unwaxed, flavored, and plain. Choose the one you're most comfortable with but, most importantly, use it! Flossing once daily is crucial to removing between-teeth plaque that your toothbrush and mouthwash can't touch. And that helps prevent gum disease.

Toothbrush. The American Dental Association (ADA) recommends brushing at least twice daily with a soft-bristled toothbrush—the head should be small enough to reach all sides of the teeth. And don't forget to brush your tongue to remove bacteria—and fight bad breath. Replace the brush every three to four months. Also consider a powered toothbrush. Sonic versions (like Sonicare) move at thirty to forty thousand strokes per minute, directing action between teeth and below the gumline.

Toothpaste. These days, you can find toothpastes and gels in just about any flavor and type imaginable. Use any formula you like, as long as it carries that ADA seal. Otherwise, you can't be sure you're getting sufficient fluoride to prevent cavities and tooth decay.

## universal truth

Talk about dedication! During visits back to Holland, Angela Visser still books appointments with her childhood dentist. And even if she can't make it back to her hometown, she's diligent about scheduling dental cleanings twice a year.

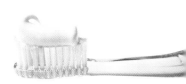

# how to get the most from a bleaching session

Whitening the teeth, whether professionally or at home, does more than make teeth look more pearly than a Mikimoto tiara. It can lend an allover glow to the entire face—and even knock a few years off your appearance. To help make sure your peroxide experience is all that it can be, heed this advice.

Know your limits. Again, not every stain can be eradicated—and some may bleach unevenly. Discuss your particular type of discoloration with your dentist to help gauge just how high your expectations should be. Also, keep in mind that bleach only works on natural teeth. If you have bonding, tooth-colored fillings, or veneers that have yellowed, they may stand out against whitened chompers.

Don't overdo it. The above applies even if you use whitening products ten times a day. Overdosing on bleaching products in pursuit of a whiter smile can be irritating to the gums and cause painful tooth sensitivity. Besides, a blindingly bright grin is almost as unflattering as a corn-kernel one—okay, maybe not quite.

Start fresh. To make sure bleach adheres and penetrates as evenly as possible, brush well first (and if possible, get a professional cleaning) before starting a whitening treatment to remove tartar and plaque buildup.

Ditch the bad habits. It hardly makes sense to spend hundreds of dollars on a power bleaching appointment if you're going to start piling on the stains the next day. No one's saying you have to completely give up the Pinot Noir and morning espresso, but consider cutting back. And be sure to brush teeth well after drinking or smoking. Indeed, many dentists say patients become much more careful about maintaining their teeth and gums after bleaching them.

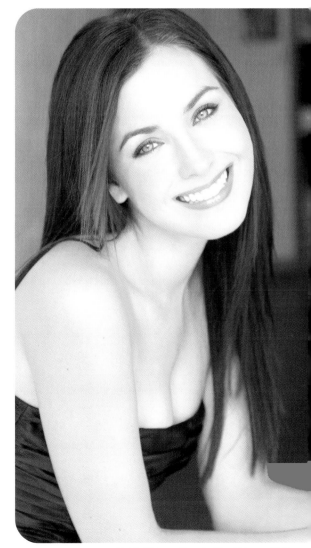

Natalie Glebova, Canada, Miss Universe 2005

# traveling right

## Brook Lee, USA, Miss Universe 1997

In her early twenties, Hawaii native Brook Lee was known as the Susan Lucci of pageants. "I never won," she says. "I would stand up there and be gracious and polite. I was a professional loser—I was good at it." At the time, all Brook cared about was scraping together enough money to put herself through college. Entering local pageants (along with hula dancing and modeling in shopping malls) seemed the most lucrative way to do it. For two straight years, she lost every contest she entered—and accumulated thousands of dollars worth of scholarships in the process. Finally, at age twenty-four, her ship came in. Brook won Miss Hawaii USA, then sailed through the Miss USA competition and moved on to Miss Universe.

If she had to name one beauty secret that helped her win the top crown, Brook would probably credit her alluring wit. "A lot of critics have said, 'She wasn't the most beautiful, but she had a way with words,'" Brook says. Indeed, her crack sense of humor and timing is still one of her most dazzling attributes. And nowhere is that more apparent than when she recalls her days traveling around the world with her Miss Universe gear in tow. "I carried a gun case with my crown in it every time I boarded an airplane," she laughs. "People in baggage claim would always stare at the case and ask what was inside. Some of them wanted to try on my crown, and of course I let them. There are pictures floating around of pilots and flight attendants wearing that crown. I figured, if I'm Miss Universe, we're all Miss Universe."

Now an actress, Brook still travels quite a bit for work. With no crown and far fewer evening gowns to take with her, globe-trotting is considerably easier. She's always careful to pack as little as possible, nearly always fitting her gear into a carry-on or two that she can easily tote herself. One thing that hasn't changed since her Miss Universe days: Brook still steps off the plane looking a little more gorgeous than the rest of us. For the scoop on how to look and feel your best when traveling, read on.

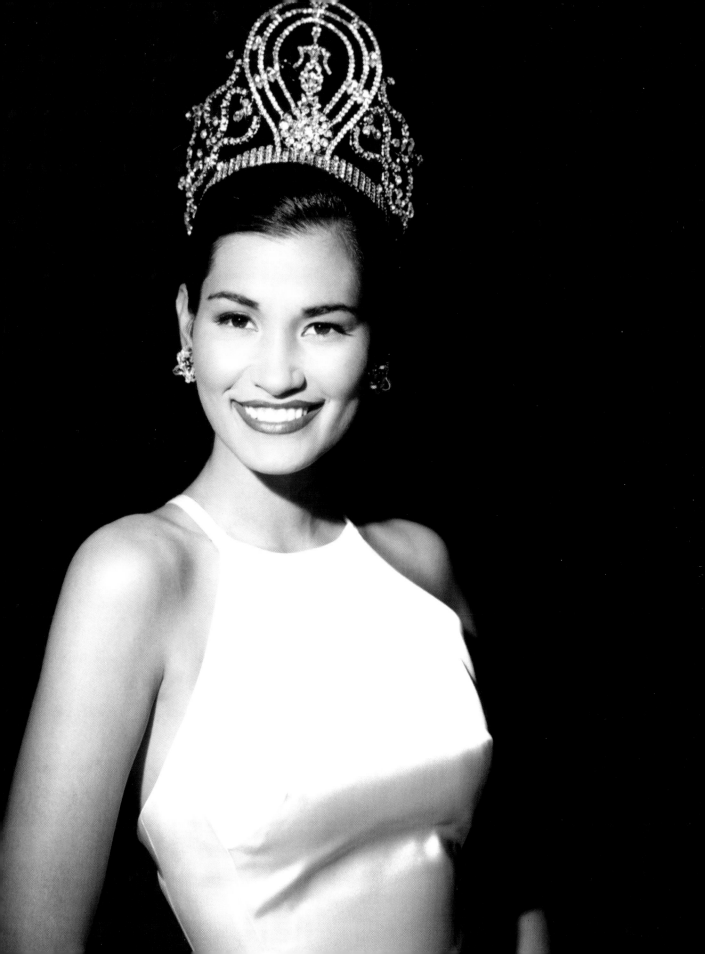

# flying right

The 2005 Miss Universe hopefuls arrived in Bangkok three weeks before the official competition—and predictably, they were mobbed by photographers the minute they landed. It's a good thing your average pageant contestant can manage to look fabulous after hours of cramped air travel, but the average woman is lucky if she can find her toiletry bag in the bottom of her carry-on. Note these pointers before you deplane.

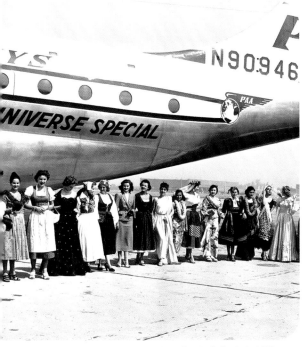

Miss Universe contestants arriving in Long Beach, California, in 1953

## Fight dehydration from the inside out.
Humidity levels inside an airplane cabin are frighteningly low, which is why even oily skin feels parched and papery by the time the landing light goes on. "Nothing helps the skin look good more than plain water," says Wendy Fitzwilliam (Trinidad & Tobago, Miss Universe 1999), who is fanatical about guzzling the stuff whether or not she's in flight. Down a bottle before taking off, then follow with at least one bottle for every hour of flying time. And resist the lure of the cocktail cart—alcohol will only dehydrate you further.

## And from the outside in.
Wendy babies her face with moisturizer before stepping on a plane. And she brings plenty of her own along for the ride—her favorite is from a line called Jencare. "The little things of lotion they give you in first class aren't enough," says the former titleholder, who totes along Neutrogena Swiss Formula for her feet and hands, reapplying lotion throughout the flight. One last line about lotion: If you're in a window seat, make sure your face and hand moisturizer contains sunscreen; damaging UV rays can travel through glass.

## Save the makeup for when you need it.
When you're slathering on lotion every hour, you don't want to slick it over a layer of foundation and powder. Keep your face as bare as possible during flight—then primp just before landing. Brook Lee's quickie pre-landing routine (the one she uses whenever she's dashing from one event to the next) is simple: "A little blush on the cheeks and gloss on the lips," she says. "It wakes you up instantly, and brings back the circulation. Then I brush on some mascara and I'm good to go."

## Help out your hair.
The low humidity inside an airplane cabin ravages more than just your skin. Even a short flight can leave your hair looking limp and lifeless—unless you're Brook Lee. She clips her tresses into a high ponytail for the duration of the trip. Not only does this keep hair out of her face, but it lifts locks at the roots. When she unclips just before landing, hair looks sleek, yet voluminous.

Air travel, of course, is only one fraction of your time away from home. Here's how to stay beautiful every day of your trip.

### Think ahead.
Wendy Fitzwilliam keeps a toiletry travel bag packed and ready to go at all times. Put together your beauty kit when you're at home and feeling relaxed, so you can plot out exactly which items you'll use while you're away. Buy enough empty plastic bottles to hold the products you'll need—many toiletry bags come with storage bottles that nestle neatly inside. And keep them three-quarters of the way full. (If you fill them all the way, they may burst or leak when exposed to heat or excessive movement.) If you take a particular prescription medication regularly, it's also a good idea to keep copies of those prescriptions in your bag at all times, in case you need an emergency refill while you're away.

### Let the hotel lend a hand.
Let's face it, we all forget *something*. (Either that, or the airline confiscates a razor or tweezers.) Before you go searching for replacements, check out the basket of goodies the hotel has left for you in the bathroom. The best hotels provide premium shampoos, lotions, and, yes, razors. If you're still short on a beauty product, very often the front desk concierge will secure it for you. (And if you don't use those mini toiletries the hotel provides, consider stashing them in your travel bag for future use.)

### Bring sleep aides.
Getting adequate sleep may just be the best beauty secret going. Unfortunately, tucking yourself into a strange bed doesn't always make for great dozing conditions—especially if you're jet-lagged. Rather than relying on sleeping pills—many of them can leave you more groggy in the morning—tote along a cushy eye mask, a small bottle of calming lavender oil to drip on your pillow, and something soothing that reminds you of home. Wendy Fitzwilliam never travels without her mini photo album, filled with snapshots of her sister, parents, boyfriend, and other loved ones. "I stand it up on my night table so I can look at it before I fall asleep," she says.

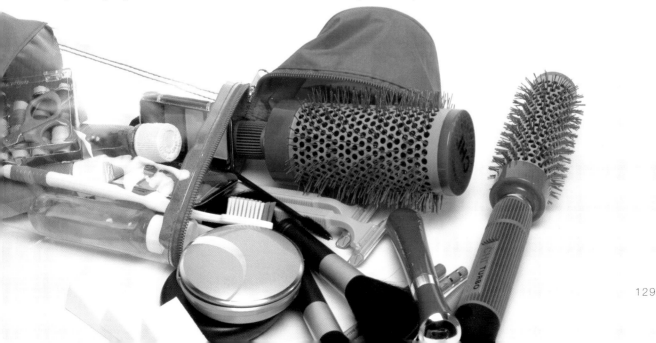

# pack less, wear more

After Justine Pasek (Panama, Miss Universe 2002) assumed the throne, she began living her life on the road, championing her official cause (HIV/AIDS prevention) in Japan, Bali, Thailand, Cambodia, Canada, and Ecuador. When you live that much of your life out of a suitcase, you'd better pack wisely. Miss Universe style gurus Billie Causieestko and David Profeta—together with a few well-traveled titleholders—offer some pointers.

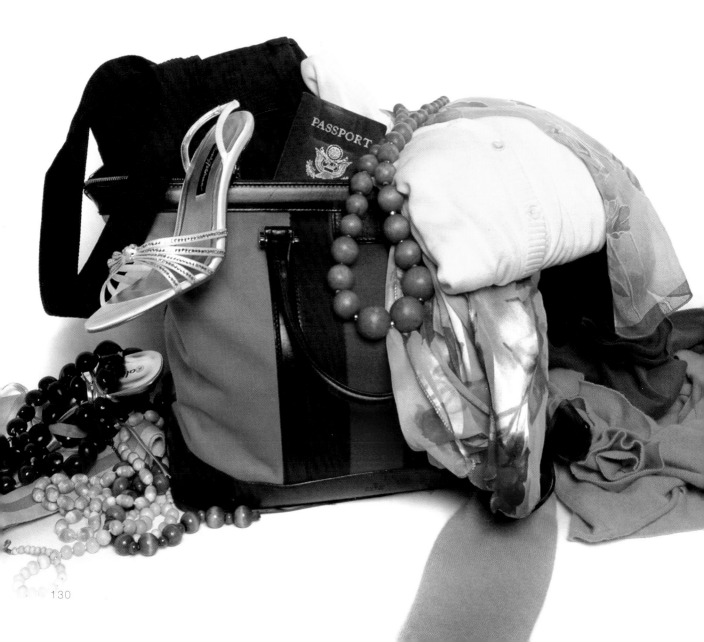

**Stash a scarf.** They scrunch easily into any suitcase pocket and offer an easy way to dress up an otherwise bland outfit or tame unruly hair. Twist one into a fabulous belt and pair it with a pair of jeans. Fold another bandana-style and use it to hold back your tresses. Or turn a large scarf into a delicate wrap for an evening cocktail party.

**Accent with accessories.** Who wants to waste space packing a different outfit for every day of the week? Natalie Glebova (Canada, Miss Universe 2005) prefers to pack extra jewelry instead. "It's amazing how you can throw on a necklace and make the simple shirt you wore two days ago look like something totally different," she says. The same goes for shoes. She brought two pairs of white capri pants for her three weeks in Bangkok in 2005. "But when I changed my shoes," she swears, "the pants took on a whole new character."

**Watch the weather.** Definitely consider the climate you're jetting off to before packing. But it's just as important to choose fabrics that will hold up when they're jammed into the back of a suitcase. Don't even attempt to tote anything linen with you unless you plan on having it pressed immediately, says Profeta. One hundred per-cent cotton is also a bad idea. Instead, choose cotton blends and knits—wrinkles tend to fall right out of them. That means light sweaters, a jersey-knit wrap dress, and skirts with a bit of stretch to them are all safe bets.

**Toss in a few more extras.** Shoes and jewelry aren't your only options when it comes to stretching your travel wardrobe. Pack a lightweight cardigan—preferably one with a bit of sparkle or beading—and use it to change the look of a simple black fitted T-shirt, Causieestko advises. "A great hat or tweed jacket will have the same effect."

**Add a bag.** Because we always seem to travel home with more clothes than we arrived with, stash a crush-able carry-on in your suitcase so that you can tote your new finds home easily.

# the jet set

Here is a look back at some of the Miss Universe Pageant's greatest moments in globe-trotting.

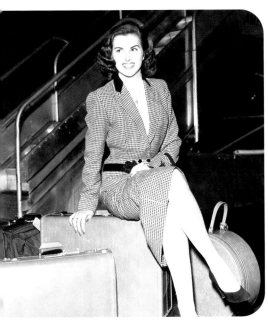

Christiane Martel, France, Miss Universe 1953

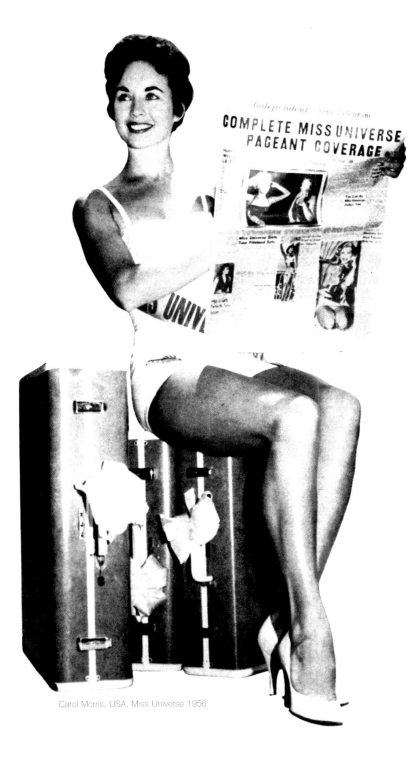

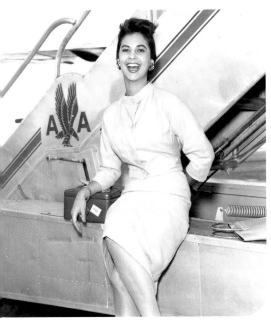

Luz Marina Zuluaga, Colombia, Miss Universe 1958

Carol Morris, USA, Miss Universe 1956

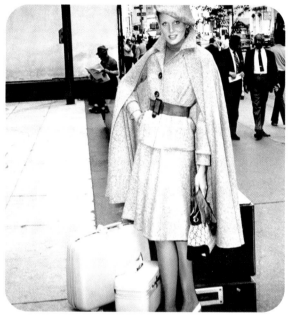

Karen Morrison, Miss USA 1974

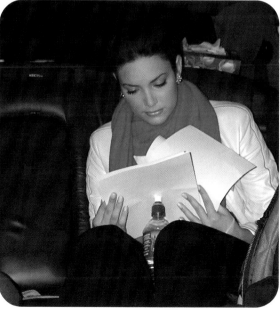

Denise M. Quiñones August, Puerto Rico, Miss Universe 2001

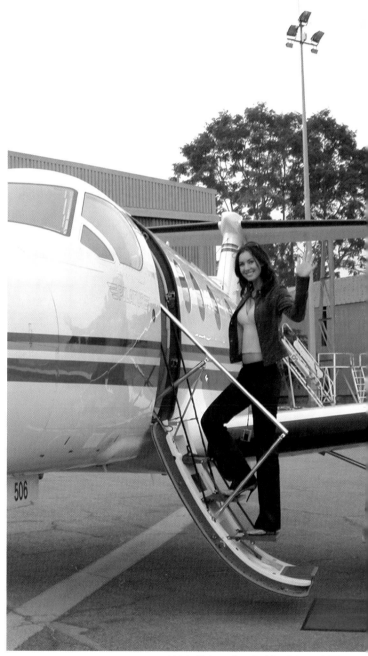

Natalie Glebova, Canada, Miss Universe 2005

# the portable workout

Just because you're on vacation doesn't mean your workout routine has to take a hiatus. To counter the hours of sitting-still time she spends during plane travel, Brook Lee uses the airport as her gym. "I never take the people movers, and I always take the stairs," she says. "It may not seem like much, but the movement really accumulates when you have to dash from the United terminal to Southwest." Also, remember that most hotels have fitness rooms and pools—and they're often blissfully empty. But if you're like Natalie Glebova, you might prefer to run through your workout in the comfort of your own hotel suite. We asked Miss Universe trainers Robert Sidbury and Clayton James (of New York's Reebok Sports Club) for some basic strength-training moves you can take anywhere.

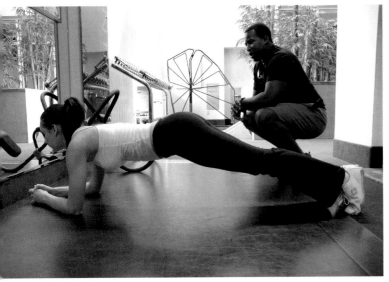

Natalie Glebova, Canada, Miss Universe 2005

The plank: Works the core muscle groups as well as shoulder stabilizers and glutes.

1. Lie on the floor, stomach down.

2. Lift your body off the ground, while keeping your forearms flat against the floor and your upper arms perpendicular to the floor so that your elbows are bent at a ninety-degree angle.

3. Lift up onto the balls of your feet so that your body is straight as a board hovering above the ground.

4. Hold for twenty seconds, building that time up to one full minute.

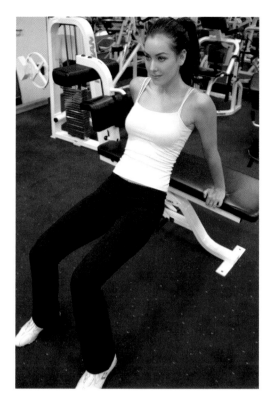

**Bench dip**: Works the triceps.

1. Rest the palms of your hands on the edge of a sturdy chair seat or bed.

2. Extend your legs in front of you so that your feet are flat on the ground, your knees are bent slightly (for a more challenging exercise, keep your legs straight in front of you), and your back is straight and close to the chair or bed throughout the motion.

3. Bend your arms so that your elbows point backward. *Slowly* lower yourself until your shoulders are at a ninety-degree angle with your elbows, then return to the starting position.

4. Repeat for two to three sets of twelve.

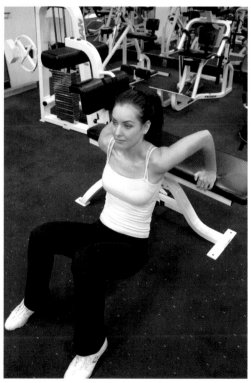

Natalie Glebova, Canada, Miss Universe 2005

## universal truth

As an adjunct to the moves on these pages, work your lower body with squats and lunges. And because cardio workouts are just as important as strength training, pack a jump rope into your suitcase and try skipping rope for one minute bursts—it's harder than you'd think! Or simply make time for daily jogs or brisk walks around your hotel's neighborhood.

# tool box

The list of travel must-haves is as individual as the trip you're taking—some people only need a pair of jeans, a backpack, and an extra T-shirt. Others (like the average Miss Universe contestant) practically require a moving truck to tote all their costumes and evening gowns. But here's a rundown of the little stuff you're most likely to forget as you're dashing to the airport. Bon voyage!

Bobby pins. Pack a stash of bobby pins in a color that matches your hair for an invisible way to smooth frizz and flyaways.

Hair rubber bands. Stow a pile of no-snag ponytail holders into your carry-on pocket. And be sure to get them in a shade that matches your hair. Throwing your locks into a sleek ponytail is one of the easiest ways to look smooth and polished in no time.

Handiwipes. Soap and water aren't always in ready supply—and a quick swab with a handiwipe is the next best thing to lathering up.

Personal stuff. Your period may not be due for another few weeks, but travel tends to rattle even the most predictable schedules, so be prepared.

Pill box. In addition to any prescription meds (and remember to carry copies of those Rx forms with you), tote a small supply of pain reliever, antacid, and an allergy cure such as Benadryl.

Sewing kit. Even if you don't sew, anyone can mend a hem or stitch a loose button. And make sure the kit includes safety pins—which suddenly come in very handy when the buckle breaks on your only pair of shoes.

Tissues. Buy a bunch of small packs of tissues and carry them everywhere. Toilet paper is practically a luxury in some public restrooms.

## universal truth

Want to make your suitcase a bit more compact? You might start with your favorite hair styling tool. Most hotels are happy to loan blow-dryers to any guest who needs one—it may not be salon-quality, but it'll do in a pinch. Or, simply air-dry your hair while you're away, using this trick: Wash or condition hair at bedtime, blot it dry, then slick on a touch of styling cream. Twist locks into three or four small braids, then go to sleep. You'll wake up with soft, smooth waves in the morning.

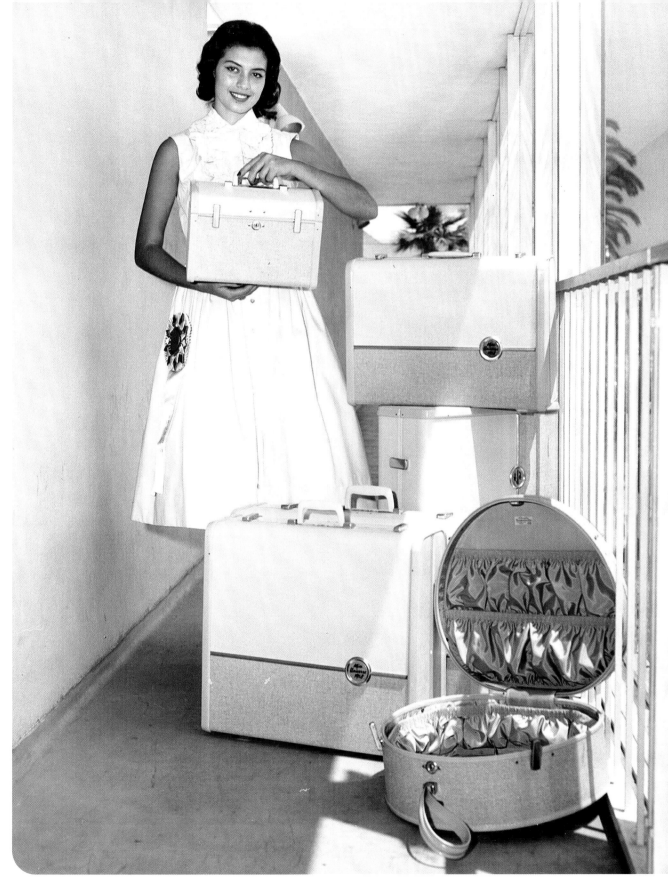

Gladys Zender, Peru, Miss Universe 1957

# how to handle a travel beauty crisis

It happens to everyone—including Miss Universe. You're stuck on unfamiliar turf when a beauty emergency strikes. What to do? If you're Natalie Glebova, you use any resource available. When she encountered a bad hair day in super-humid Bangkok during the three weeks of competitions leading up to the Miss Universe Pageant, she was lucky enough to have a supply of headbands and scarves tucked into her suitcase. Voilá, suddenly that misbehaving mane is one magnificent style! Below, some other common travel crises and how to cope.

## ooops! a stain

Stains come in all shapes, sizes, and types. But one thing they have in common: The sooner you can get them out, the better.

**Blot it out.** If you're dealing with a liquid, grab a clean cloth (many stylists swear by baby wipes in emergencies) and firmly pat the stained area to remove the excess. Don't rub—you'll only set the stain further. If you've spilled something non-liquid on your clothes, start by scraping off whatever you can with a butter knife.

**Cool it down.** If you can remove the stained clothing, bring it to a faucet and flush the soiled spot with cold water. (Hot temperatures can set stains.) If this isn't possible, dunk a towel in a bowl of ice water so that it's soaking wet, then blot the stain again.

**Pretreat.** If you've brought a pretreating detergent stick with you, apply it to the stain. If not, try to have the clothing laundered within the next twenty-four hours.

**Use caution.** Can't have the garment cleaned for another week? There's still hope of saving the item. Just don't have it ironed or pressed until you've had a chance to remove the soiling—again, heat may set the stain. And when you finally are able to wash it, pretreat the area first to increase the chances that the stain will lift out.

## whoa, you look tired

If jet leg has left you feeling like a zombie and looking even worse, it's time to bring your face back to life.

**Please your peepers.** Clear bloodshot eyes with a few drops of Visine—getting the red out is more than half the battle.

**Line your eyes.** Apply a beige or taupe liner along the inner rims of the eyes to brighten them.

**Put away the pinks.** Eye shadows in the pink family will magnify any redness in or around the eyes. Instead, stick with pale neutral shadows, like beige and pale gray.

**Be a curl friend.** Curling your lashes will make your eyes look more open instantly.

**Get a glow.** No matter how rushed or tired you are in the morning, don't forget the blush. Exhaustion tends to make the healthiest complexion look pallid—a pop of rosy pink on the apples of your cheeks can make all the difference.

# last night's dinner didn't agree with you

Okay, so this isn't exactly a beauty dilemma—unless you consider that your post-feast indigestion is written all over your face! Here's how to deal with a queasy stomach, nausea, and other unmentionables.

**Stop eating.** You probably won't want to eat anyway. Stay away from solid foods for at least four hours to allow your stomach a chance to settle.

**Take your meds.** While you're waiting for your gut to calm down, take an antacid such as Pepto-Bismol.

**Start with liquids.** If you're experiencing vomiting or diarrhea, stay off the solid foods for the day. But keep the body hydrated with lots of clear fluids. Sip water, ginger ale, bouillon, and weak tea. But avoid anything containing dairy, which could further upset your stomach.

**Try the solid stuff.** If you're still feeling icky on day two, continue to steer clear of anything fatty or milk-based. Instead, choose dry toast, plain rice, bananas, and canned fruit. On day three, you can move on to lean meats, boiled eggs, and potatoes.

Natalie Glebova
Canada, Miss Universe 2005

**Seek help.** Still little improvement by the end of day four? Find a local clinic and get a doctor's checkup.

**Think ahead.** Next time you're away, remember a few basics: If there are warnings about eating unwashed fruit or drinking local water, heed them—even if it means brushing your teeth with the bottled stuff and avoiding all ice in drinks.

# neither did the exotic drinks

During her travels Miss Universe is the honored guest at many diplomatic functions. Unfortunately, in some countries that means many toasts are offered in her honor. When you're hung over, no amount of makeup or hair product can change that. But help is on the way!

**Have another drink.** And we're not talking about hair of the dog. Guzzle a full glass of water as soon as you wake up. Alcohol is severely dehydrating—that awful headache is largely your body's cry for $H_2O$.

**Take a pill.** Knock out the headache extra fast by popping a couple of aspirin or other pain reliever first thing in the morning. Pain relievers containing caffeine may be slightly more helpful—but just remember that the stimulant will further dehydrate you. So keep guzzling water.

**Eat the right stuff.** Hangover cravings tend to fall into two camps—you either want a fat-laden egg sandwich or nothing at all. The best bet falls somewhere in between. Eat a breakfast rich in vitamins—especially vitamin C, which your body loses during a night of drinking. A fruit salad paired with a soothing bowl of oatmeal is ideal.

**Hit the hay.** It may seem like a waste to spend a day in bed, but a few extra hours of shut-eye will help the body restore itself in time for the evening. Just try to take it easy this time, okay?

# teen beauty

## Allie LaForce, Miss Teen USA 2005

When Allie LaForce won the Miss Teen USA crown in August 2005, she entered a world of television appearances, celebrity sightings, fabulous clothes, and all the CoverGirl cosmetics she could ever want. Did the high school junior from Vermillion, Ohio, morph into an evening gown–wearing junior diva overnight? Not a chance.

Allie has always felt most at home on the basketball court and softball field. And when she's not playing games, she's rooting on the sidelines. "I love watching football," she gushes. "My family has Browns season tickets."  But just because this self-described jock enjoys a good sweaty scuffle doesn't mean she doesn't embrace her girly side, too. "I don't understand why people think you can't be a lady and do sports at the same time," says Allie, who counts the stunning WNBA star Lisa Leslie as one of her idols.

Allie's approach to beauty is always low-key and low-maintenance, even when she's rubbing shoulders with A-listers at special events. "I'm very natural," she says. "I barely wear any makeup. Just mascara and lip gloss, which I pretty much have on 24/7." Her gloss of choice: CoverGirl Wetslicks in Peaches and Gleam, which she describes as "a light pink frost color—it's not sticky or too thick, so my hair doesn't stick to it." As for those gorgeous blonde tresses of hers, however, Allie admits the upkeep isn't completely effortless. "I have a big old thick mane of hair, so it takes me a good twenty-five minutes to blow-dry it," she says. Sounds like a sport in itself!

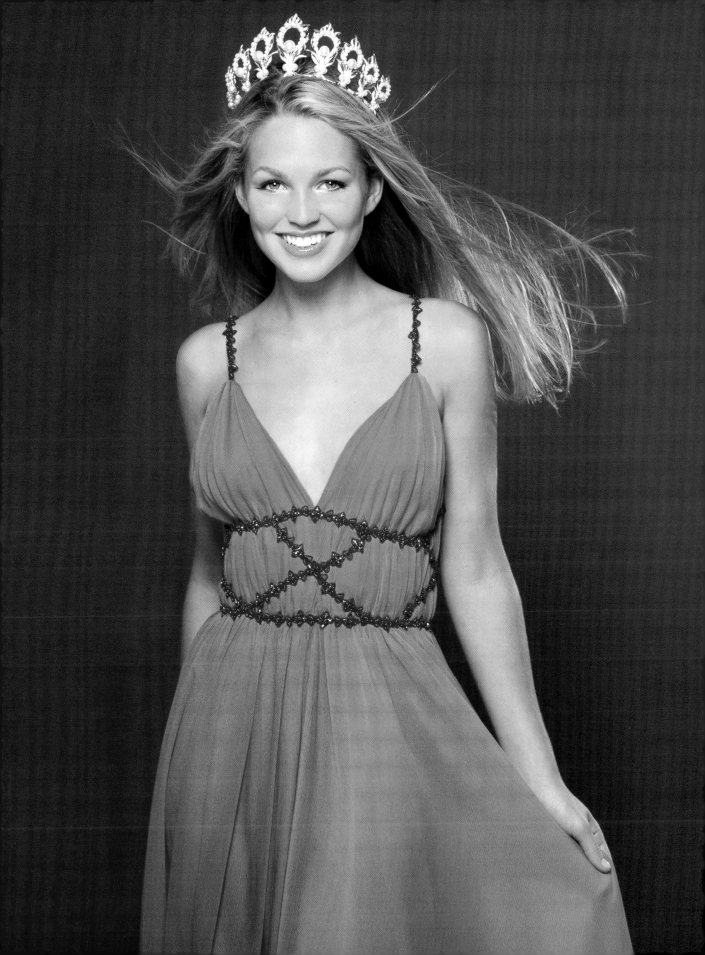

# face time

Aside from the $12,000 Mikimoto tiara she has stashed at home, Shelley Hennig (Miss Teen USA, 2004) isn't too different from your average teenager. She takes tap dance lessons, makes silly videos with her friends—and gets the occasional pimple. "I don't break out very often, but when I do get a pimple, it's a biggie," she says.

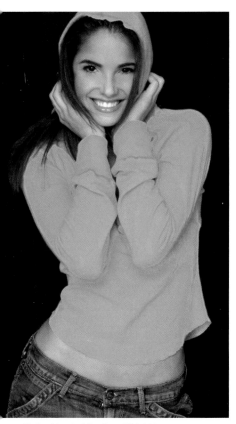

Shelley Hennig, Miss Teen USA 2004

## acne s.o.s.

It seems like just yesterday when you barely knew the meaning of the term *zit*. Now you're scanning your face for spots in every mirror you pass. As any high school grad can attest, even the most well-behaved, baby-smooth skin can turn angry and rebellious—usually at the worst moments! But don't take it personally—those breakouts are your body's way of telling you it's going through major changes. Before you get angry, get informed.

**Hormones start hopping.** Puberty brings on more than just menstruation and womanly curves. It also causes a release of hormones called androgens, which sends your skin's oil glands (or pores) into high gear—that's why nearly all teens have oily skin. The most active oil glands are located around your forehead, nose, and chin (the T-zone), so pores may look larger in those areas and skin may become shiny minutes after you've washed your face. Not to worry, once your body settles down, the oil production will, too.

**Skin starts shedding.** Around this time, the skin cells inside your pores begin to shed more rapidly than ever before—and mix with the increased amount of oil your body is producing. Together, the skin cells and oil form a sticky substance that can easily clog pores, causing—you guessed it—blackheads and whiteheads.

**Those bumps get angry.** We all have bacteria growing on our skin. But sometimes it gets so cozy inside a clogged pore that it starts multiplying like crazy. That's how a tiny zit turns into a monster one.

## universal truth

For Shelley Hennig, Clean & Clear acne gel keeps most breakouts at bay. But she does recall waking up one morning—a few hours before she was about to leave for the Miss Teen USA Pageant in Palm Springs—to a very unpleasant surprise: "I had a big zit on my forehead," she says. "I went straight to the dermatologist, she injected it, and it went away." The dermatologist is the one person who is allowed to poke and prod your pimples. Using sterilized equipment, a doctor can treat zits with a shot of special steroids, which usually makes the bump vanish within a day or two. This is an especially good treatment for cyst-like pimples, which can take weeks to clear up—and often leave a scar behind.

# don't freak!

We know, it's difficult not to stress when that bump on your chin feels bigger than Mount Everest. But worrying about your breakouts could make them worse. To the rescue—a slew of super-powered pimple products!

## what to do

**Start at the drugstore.** If you're only getting the occasional zit, over-the-counter remedies might work just fine. After washing with a mild cleanser, try a gentle, alcohol-free toner containing salicylic acid (which breaks down the dead skin cells inside the pores), followed by a spot treatment with benzoyl peroxide (which attacks bacteria and dries up oil).

**Upgrade your zit creams.** For more stubborn acne, you should see a dermatologist, who can help design a better plan of attack. Cheryl Thellman-Karcher, the dermatologist who has been treating reigning Miss Teen USAs for years, usually starts her younger patients on a more concentrated form of benzoyl peroxide, along with other creams designed to zap away bacteria before it can invade your pores. If those don't work, topical products containing retinoids usually do. Retinoids help fight inflammation and open pores—which means they help calm current zits while preventing new ones.

**Fight 'em from the inside out.** Still not seeing results? Your dermatologist might prescribe antibiotic pills to wipe out the bacteria the lotions can't kill. Some doctors also put teens on oral contraceptives to keep those wacky hormones in check. And in extreme cases, your dermatologist may suggest a medication called Accutane, which dramatically slows down oil production by shrinking the oil glands. Accutane has some pretty serious side effects; it's very important to discuss all of them with your doc.

## what not to do

**Panic.** Once again, stress only spells trouble for acne. First off, some experts believe it increases oil production. Second, the more you worry, the more you're likely to nervously poke at your face. And that brings us to . . .

**Pick.** We know that zit is screaming out to be popped, but resist the urge. Attempting to operate on a pimple can lead to permanent scarring and infection (because who knows what's under your fingernails?). And the harder you squeeze, the more you risk forcing the stuff inside the blemish deeper under the skin.

**Overdose.** When you want a breakout gone yesterday, it's tempting to start loading up on every acne cleanser and cream in the drugstore. Bad idea, says Thellman-Karcher. Most of these products are pretty harsh, so using more than one or two at a time can leave even oily skin red, irritated, and slow to clear. If you're unsure exactly how much your face can handle, check with a dermatologist. And forget grainy scrubs—they may make you feel cleaner, but the scratchy particles in most of them can open up pimples, causing more infection and possible scarring.

**Try sketchy treatments.** There are tons of so-called natural remedies out there. The problem: There's no proof that they work, and many of them (especially those essential oils) may make your acne worse. Steer clear of them.

**Go on a diet.** We've all heard the rumors that chocolate and fried foods make acne worse. But again, no one's ever proved a connection. Of course, if you notice a flare-up every time you eat a Hershey bar, it might be wise to cut back and see if your breakouts improve.

**Use oily hair products.** If your spots are concentrated around your forehead and hairline, your styling products may be the culprit. If you have bangs or long hair that falls in your face, your oily creams and serums can migrate onto the skin, clogging the pores. Also, consider your sleep habits. If you doze with one cheek on a pillowcase that's already saturated with hair product residue, you could be pressing the stuff into your skin. Try tying your hair back at bedtime and washing pillowcases often.

# three simple steps to seriously amazing skin

Of course, one of the best ways to fight pimples is to prevent them from erupting in the first place. And that starts with good skin care. Shelley Hennig never, ever goes to bed with makeup on. "I always wash my face morning and night," she says. Because her skin is on the drier side, Shelley's diligent about moisturizing her face and neck at bedtime. Sure, it might be a drag to slog through your skin care routine morning and night—but the good news is that, at this age there's no need to bother with a complex regime of creams and potions. Just cleanse, protect, and dahling, you look like a million bucks!

Wash up. For most teens, the best cleanser is gentle, mild, and oil-free. Unless your skin is very dry (which is unlikely), avoid creamy formulas, and choose one that's either clear or foaming. And even if you have acne, it's usually a good idea to avoid medicated cleansers, which can strip the skin of the essential oils it needs to stay healthy. Washing with very hot water will also strip away those good oils. So start by rinsing with tepid water, then massage your cleanser into the face using smaller circular motions with the tips of your fingers. (Don't bother using a washcloth—it's too abrasive and can harbor pimple-causing bacteria.) Rinse again with tepid water, splashing until skin no longer feels slick or slippery.

Moisturize. Contrary to popular belief, moisturizer doesn't prevent wrinkles, so use it only where you actually need it. After patting your face dry, apply a dot of oil-free lotion on dry or rough areas. If those spots still feel flaky or parched, add a bit more—or try switching to a slightly richer moisturizer.

Protect. Want to truly prevent wrinkles? Sunscreen is truly the best age cream out there. Wearing an SPF 15 or higher *every time* you go outside (even if it's just sitting in a car or walking to school) will help shield you from the sun's ultraviolet light—the same light that winds up causing wrinkles, sagging, skin cancer, and other not-so-fun stuff years from now. Start getting serious about your sunscreen today, and you'll be one sizzling lady later on.

## universal truth

Most acne creams are best used at night because they can make skin more sensitive to the sun—and because some creams become less effective when exposed to light. If using a moisturizer in addition to an acne product, apply the medicated product first, then wait ten minutes and rub on a light coat of moisturizer. If your doctor has told you to use the zit cream in the morning, wear it underneath your sunscreen.

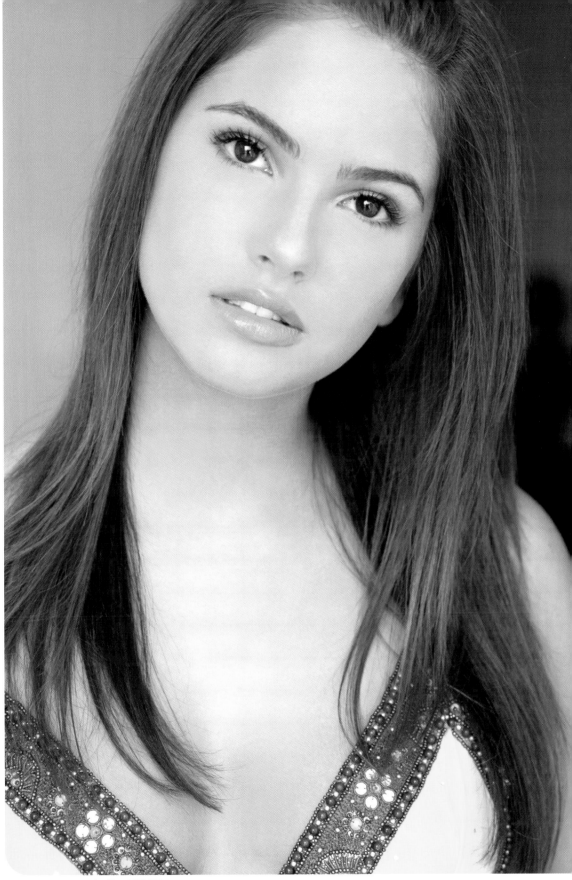

Shelley Hennig, Miss Teen USA 2004

# mad about makeup

Dealing with school, parents, and dating dramas is heavy enough without your makeup weighing you down, too. Foundation, eye shadow, and mascara look prettiest when you can barely tell you're wearing them. "I always like more natural styles for teens that are a little fun," says Linda Rondinella-Osgood, who has coordinated the hair and makeup for Miss Teen USA since 1995. "Sometimes girls wind up covering up their natural beauty, and that's a shame."

## your skin, only better

First things first: If you're one of those rare birds who has barely had a blemish in her life, you can stop reading right now. Your skin is at its absolute best right now, and it would be a crime not to show it off. These days, the coolest way to wear foundation, powder, and concealer is to smooth them only over red or blemished spots—not to coat the entire face like a mask. But if you need a little help, read on.

Take the tint. Tinted moisturizer is an excellent choice for anyone who has good skin, but feels naked without a little something on top. These dream creams warm up and smooth the complexion without smothering it. And because they're super-sheer, you don't have to worry about matching your skin tone precisely—just try to get as close a match as possible.

Go a bit heavier—but not too much. If you do choose to wear a true foundation, don't just dip into your mom's toiletry bag. Adult makeup is typically too heavy and pore-clogging for teens. Look for oil-free, slightly watery formulas that you can easily shake in the bottle. Those will look the sheerest and most natural—and won't cause acne.

Find your perfect match. Another reason not to steal Mom's makeup: Foundation should match your skin so well that it practically melts into your face, so you should test formulas on your own skin before buying. If you're at a department store counter with tester bottles, swab three shades along your jaw-line to see which matches best. If you can't open the bottle, holding it up to your chin will give you a pretty good idea of its match potential.

Earn extra credit. Why just cover the skin when you can make it healthier? Many foundations contain acne medications to help clear blemishes while disguising them. Others have a little bit of sunscreen—but because it's usually not enough to fully protect the face from the sun, be sure to wear a separate SPF formula underneath your makeup.

Get powder power. Powder comes in two forms: loose (which is great for setting your foundation) and pressed (which comes in a compact and can be a great substitute for foundation). Both forms leave the skin with a polished, matte finish—and can be especially useful in shiny areas. Keep in mind that if you do powder your face, it's best to use only powdered blush and eye shadow along with it because creamy formulas will turn pasty.

Keep it clean. Makeup brushes, sponges, and especially your own fingers are breeding grounds for pimple-causing germs. Wash those sponges and brushes at least once a week with an antibacterial soap—and always lather up your hands before bringing them anywhere near your face.

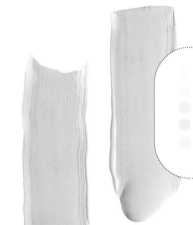

## universal truth

Beware of ultra-dark eye pencils—and especially liquid liner. Both can make the eyes look ultra-tiny and give the entire face an Elvira vibe. If you want to define the eyes, smudge a little brown shadow along the upper and lower lash lines for a softer look.

## color cues

Rondinella-Osgood maps out the makeup looks for Miss Teen USA with an eye toward the current trends. She may try out a funky shade of lipstick, a sizzling silver eye shadow, or a daring shot of raspberry blush on the cheeks. One of the true joys of being a teen is that you can get away with pretty much anything—up to a point. Below, some secrets to making the most of your makeup palette, without looking like a clown.

### Do some research.

Certain types of makeup go in and out of style just like clothes. (Just think of those old pictures of your mom wearing frosty blue eye shadow.) Rondinella-Osgood always incorporates the current looks when working on Miss Teen USA. "We might do retro 1960s, natural, or whatever is happening right now," she says. You can tap into the latest makeup trends by reading your favorite beauty magazines or taking a good look at a classmate whose style you admire.

### Make it your own.

Experimenting with makeup is one of the easiest ways to craft an individualized style—because, hey, if you hate it, you can wash it all off and start again. Once you have a good sense of what looks are going on now, play around at your bathroom mirror—department store makeup counters are also a great place to experiment.

### Shine on.

Metallic makeup is huge right now and shows no sign of going any-where. A dash of bronze shadow on the lids or a swipe of silver highlighting cream along the tops of the cheekbones looks sophisticated and fun at the same time.

### Keep it light.

The trick to having fun without looking funny: First, stick with sheer colors. A bright blush won't seem like war paint if it's an ultra-light gel formula. On the mouth, you can get away with a fuchsia or even orange shade if you choose a gloss over a full-bodied lipstick. Second, select only one feature to play up (the bright blush or the fuchsia lip gloss or the bronze eye shadow), and keep the rest of the face nearly bare.

# night right

For a dressed-up look, play up the eyes with a wash of silver over the lids and a dark gray contour in the crease. For the mouth, try a pale pink lipstick with a dab of golden gloss in the center. Finally, brush a bit of blush along the apples of the cheeks.

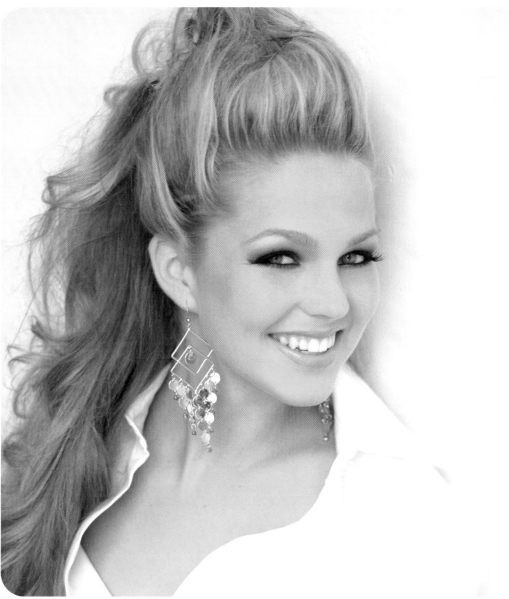

Allie LaForce, Miss Teen USA 2005

# day dreamy

When it comes to your daytime look, remember the three Fs: flirty, fun, and fresh. A pale pink gloss on the lips, paired with a touch of rosy blush swirled over the apples of the cheeks adds a just-kissed look to the face. Eyes look prettiest when you open them up with a light coat of mascara and a smudge of gray, brown, or deep eggplant shadow along the lash line.

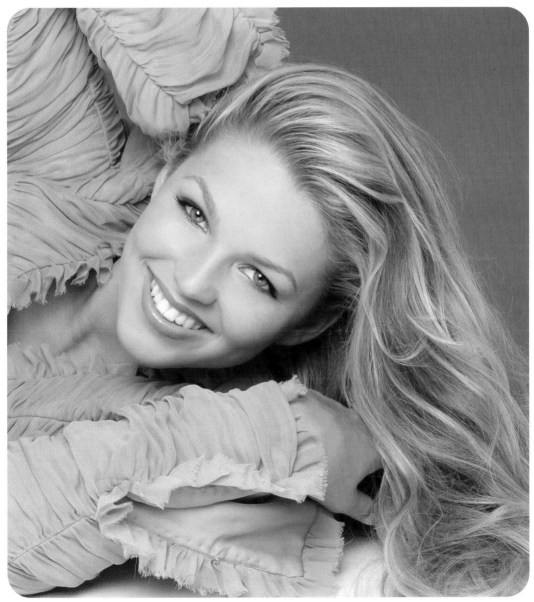

Allie LaForce, Miss Teen USA 2005

# teen queens

Ruth Zakarian was crowned the very first Miss Teen USA back in 1983, proving that young women know plenty about beauty, style, and sophistication. Here is an illustrated history of some of our favorite looks.

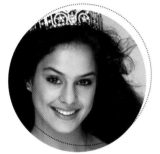
Ruth Zakarian
Miss Teen USA 1983

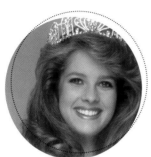
Cherise Haugen
Miss Teen USA 1984

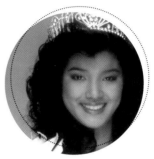
Kelly Hu
Miss Teen USA 1985

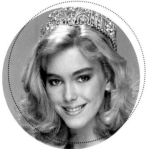
Allison Brown
Miss Teen USA 1986

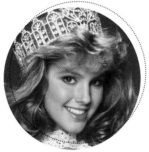
Kristi Addis
Miss Teen USA 1987

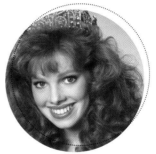
Mindy Duncan
Miss Teen USA 1988

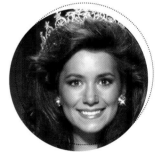
Brandi Sherwood
Miss Teen USA 1989

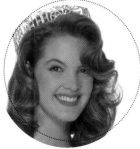
Bridgette Wilson
Miss Teen USA 1990

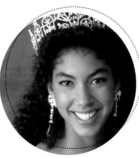
Janel Bishop
Miss Teen USA 1991

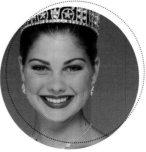
Jamie Solinger
Miss Teen USA 1992

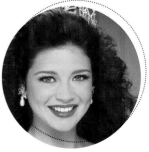
Charlotte Lopez
Miss Teen USA 1993

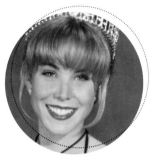

Shauna Gambill
Miss Teen USA 1994

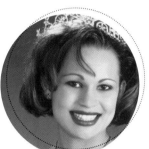

Keylee Sue Sanders
Miss Teen USA 1995

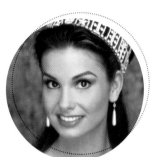

Christie Woods
Miss Teen USA 1996

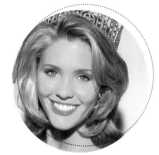

Shelly Moore
Miss Teen USA 1997

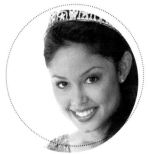

Vanessa Minnillo
Miss Teen USA 1998

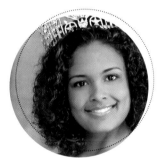

Ashley Coleman
Miss Teen USA 1999

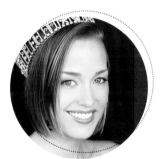

Jillian Parry
Miss Teen USA 2000

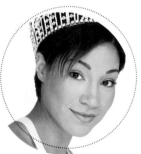

Marissa Whitley
Miss Teen USA 2001

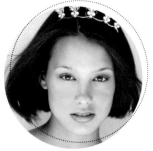

Vanessa Semrow
Miss Teen USA 2002

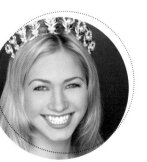

Tami Farrell
Miss Teen USA 2003

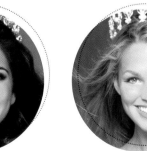

Shelley Hennig
Miss Teen USA 2004

Allie LaForce
Miss Teen USA 2005

# hot hair

New York hairstylist John Barrett, of the John Barrett Salon, adores styling hair for Miss Teen USA. That's because your high school years are when your tresses are at their absolute best. For one thing, your body's increase in oil production (the same increase that brings on acne) makes the hair more lustrous than ever. Add to that the fact that young hair hasn't gone through the harsh chemical treatments (and aging process) that older tresses have. "I've frequently had clients bring in their daughters and say, 'I want my hair to look like that—silkier, shinier, thicker,'" says Barrett. If you're not loving your hair quite as much as you should, here's how to start.

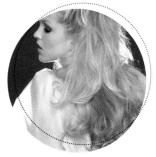

Allie LaForce
Miss Teen USA 2005

## universal truth

Miss Teen USA 2004 Shelley Hennig hates dealing with her hair so much that sometimes she wishes she were bald! Fortunately, she's found a solution that saves her from the daily grind of styling her hair. "I go to bed with it soaking wet," she says. Come morning, she wakes up to smooth waves. She enhances the shine with a bit of BioSilk Serum from Farouk, then spritzes the roots with a volumizing spray. Pretty good—pretty fast!

**Clean it correctly.** That means using the right shampoo and conditioner for your hair. For very oily tresses, use a shampoo you can see through, then apply a light conditioner (it should pour easily when you turn the bottle upside down), avoiding the inch of hair closest to your scalp, and rinse thoroughly. For drier or very thick, frizzy hair, use a creamy shampoo, then comb in a rich, soupy conditioner until all your strands—especially the ends—are coated.

**Then take the day off.** "Teen girls should not wash their hair more than twice a week," says Barrett. Relax—it's not as icky as it sounds. Rinse the hair as you normally would during your morning shower to remove excess grime, then slick on your conditioner, and rinse. Tresses will be noticeably silkier and less frizzy immediately. If you have very oily or fine hair, try cleansing your tresses every other day.

**Invest in good styling products.** We know you're not made of money. But if you're going to spend your bucks on something hair-related, better to skimp on the shampoo and pony up for a styling product that really makes your hair feel and look awesome. Using a cream or mousse that doesn't agree with your hair is just begging for a bad hair day.

**Know the difference.** Gels and mousses are best if your hair is very greasy, while styling creams combine moisture with gentle hold. Silicone serums coat strands with a slippery plastic-like substance, adding immediate shine.

**Be a little stingy.** If you think your hair is naturally limp or dull, it may just be suffering from styling-aid overdose. More than a couple drops of silicone serum can have the opposite of its intended effect, leaving a heavy, dull buildup on the hair. As for other products, start with a dime-sized blob of gel or cream or a palmful of mousse, distribute it evenly through your hair, then add more only if necessary.

**Turn down the heat.** Blow-dryers have always had multiple heat settings; now the latest flat irons and curling irons do, too. "The last generation of irons got very, very hot," says Barrett. "And that can be damaging to the hair. Now, the good ones have temperature controls. Set it to medium and you'll save your hair."

# shades of difference

Not long ago, professional hair color was strictly for grownups who either felt like shelling out big bucks for a head of highlights—or desperately needed to cover their gray. Not anymore, notes William Howe, the colorist for Miss Teen USA. "Many of them have their color done," he says. And it's not just pageant types. "A lot of average young girls are coming in. Often, they'll get just a few highlights for a drop of added brightness around the face." Yup, it's true: A subtle change in color can be enough to change your whole look—and you don't always have to pay a lot to reap the rewards.

Salon highlights. They're not exactly cheap, but you'll be paying a lot less than someone like your mom, who probably has her base shade colored along with a head full of highlights. When you're young, your hair is gray-free and in great condition. So save your tresses—and your wallet—by adding just three or four well-placed highlights to bring a new radiance to your complexion.

At-home highlights. These kits are great if you have a steady hand and don't care about getting absolutely perfect results. The lightened pieces will probably be a bit wider than the professional kind, and you may not be able to place them exactly where you want. But it gets a lot easier if you enlist a buddy to help you out.

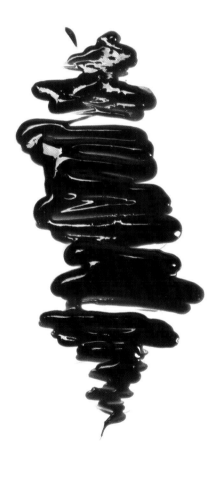

Home rinses. The term *rinse* usually refers to those drugstore box kits that fade away anywhere from several days to a few weeks after you apply them. Rinses are typically ammonia- and peroxide-free. True, that means they won't make your hair any lighter, but the good news is that they won't damage the hair. And teen hair is *super* vulnerable to harsh ingredients. What's more, rinses are low-commitment—so you can feel free to play with the wilder side of the spectrum.

Henna. Henna is a natural dye that adds golden, red, or burgundy tones to the hair. The result can be beautifully striking, if you get the color right. But it's usually very difficult to know precisely which shade your hair will turn—and if you get the color wrong, you may be stuck with it. Henna dyes can be very difficult to remove—and certain formulas turn funny colors when they're exposed to chlorine and other elements. The bottom line: Use at your own risk.

Pure peroxide. Just because women have been lightening their hair with hydrogen peroxide for years doesn't mean it's a good idea. Once you apply it, you open the hair cuticle and have no control over the bleaching action, warns Howe. If you're going to do it, he suggests mixing the peroxide with a little conditioner and combing it into small sections of the hair for homemade highlights. The conditioner will dilute the peroxide and help keep the hair from drying out.

# two easy updos

Few styles blend simplicity and sleek sophistication like a ponytail. To ensure that yours doesn't make you look like you've just walked out of gym class, start by rubbing a speck of styling cream between your palms and slicking it over dry hair. Use either a brush (for a smooth look) or your hands (for a fuller look) to gather your locks into a ponytail just below the crown of the head, and secure with a snag-free elastic. Take a tiny section of the tail, and wind it around the elastic so that it's no longer visible. Tuck the end of the section into the base of the ponytail. Fasten any flyaways firmly against the head with bobby pins that match your hair. To give your tail a polished wave, wrap it around a large Velcro roller for fifteen minutes.

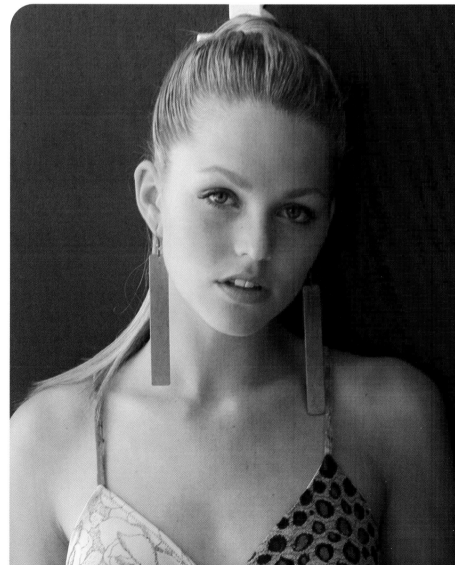

Allie LaForce, Miss Teen USA 2005

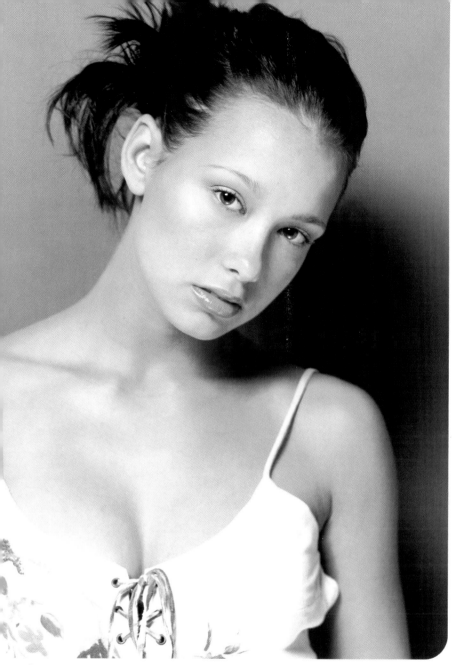

nessa Semrow, Miss Teen USA 2002

The messy ballerina bun is one of John Barrett's favorite styles—because it's just a bit wild and just a bit innocent. Skip any styling products, and start by twisting dried hair into a loose bun an inch below the crown of the head. Secure it with a snag-proof elastic band. Then, using either your fingers or the pointy end of a comb, pull several tiny pieces out of the bun. Then place the palms of your hands on the top front of your head and begin massaging until hair looks slightly mussed around your face.

# you've got the look

When Shelley Hennig was growing up, her personal style was half tomboy, half princess. On some days, her favorite accessory was a backward G.I. Joe baseball cap. On others, it was a girly pocketbook. Since then, her look has evolved into a healthy cross between fashion-conscious and downright fun. We should all take a cue from Shelley's book, says Miss Teen USA stylist Billie Causieestko. "When you're young, you have a lot of freedom to show off your individual style," she believes. "And this is the time when you have time to be a little crafty and creative with your clothes. Just make sure not to overdo it—or whatever you're wearing will stop being fashionable."

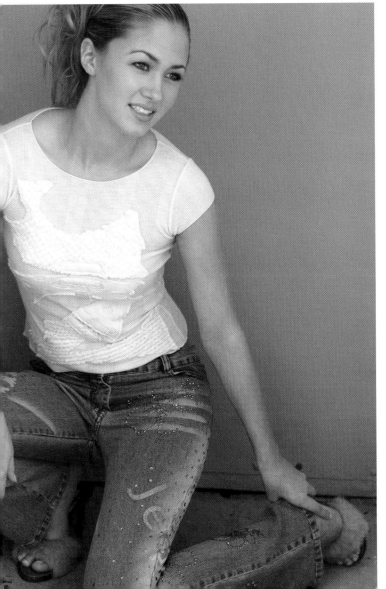

Tami Farrell, Miss Teen USA 2003

**Learn your jean-eology.** Teen trends come and go like Hollywood romances, but one seems here to stay: "Denim isn't going anywhere," says Causieestko. Invest in one pair of jeans you really love and we promise you'll be able to wear them next season.

**Get crafty.** If you do get sick of your jeans or other standbys in six months, change them! "Rhinestone your jeans or skirt. Tie ribbons to the side of your purse or attach a funky pin," says Causieestko. What a great way to get mega mileage out of your favorite stuff—and to craft a totally unique look.

**Make it your own.** That tailored tweed jacket you saw at the thrift store isn't as uptight as it looks. Sew a fun floral patch over the elbow or add a brooch to the lapel—and everyone will be dying to know where you shop!

**Tighten up.** Warm up your legs—and heat up your look—with a funky pair of opaque tights under a basic monochromatic skirt.

**Bet on brown.** Next time you have a fancy-schmancy affair to attend, swap the head-to-toe black ensemble for a chocolate brown outfit. Sophisticated yet soft—and much more flattering against teenage skin.

## the not list

When you're young, you can get away with wearing pretty much anything, except . . .

A plunging neckline—too vulgar

Any skirt or dress you have to hold when you bend over—too cheap

Traditional pantyhose—too mom-ish

Anything you wouldn't be caught dead in around your parents—too tacky

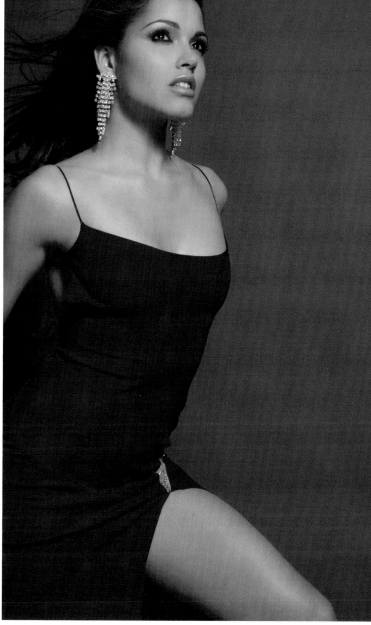

Susie Castillo, Miss USA 2003

## universal truth

How to be creative with your wardrobe without screaming "Fashion Victim"? If you're going to flaunt a killer pair of shoes or rhinestoned jeans, let those be the focal point, and keep the rest of your outfit low-key.

# tool box

You're not a little kid anymore, so if you're still working with the style supplies you used in middle school, perhaps we can suggest some upgrades.

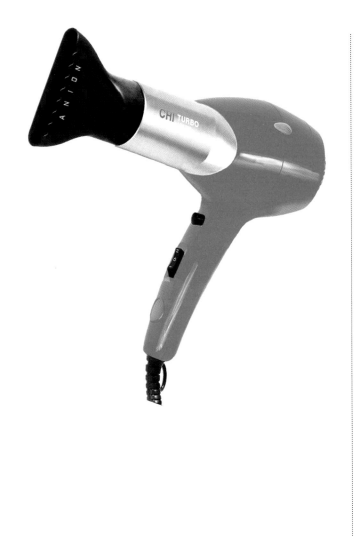

Blow-dryer. If you're still using a mini blow-dryer every morning, perhaps it's time you move up in the world. Look for one that has three settings (high, medium, and cool) and at least 1,500 watts of power.

Lip gloss. Put away the fruity stuff you've been using since third grade, and look for a long-lasting gloss that glides over the lips without feeling sticky or pasty.

Hair accessories. Enough with the scrunchies and banana clips. Replace those middle school relics with a sophisticated tortoise-shell style barrette, a few colorful scarves, and a pack of skinny hair elastics. Trés chic!

Shoes. No need to spend zillions of dollars to treat your tootsies right. But once you hit high school, those ratty old Keds don't always cut the mustard. Aim to have at least two unscuffed sets of shoes—a dark pair for winter and a lighter pair for summer—that you can wear for job interviews and other important events.

Skin regime. It's time to stop lathering your face with that bar of Ivory in the shower. Invest in a mild facial cleanser, an oil-free moisturizer, and SPF 15 sunscreen— and start using them, pronto.

# how to get gorgeous
# on the cheap

One of the major perks of winning Miss Teen USA is that you're flooded with freebies ranging from shoes to gowns to bucketloads of lipstick. Does that mean the rest of us have to drain our piggybanks to look good? No way!

**Shop seasonally.** Resist trying to replenish your wardrobe when all the new arrivals are hitting the stores. Instead, aim to buy most of your summer clothes in July and your winter gear in November. You'll find markdowns galore.

**Be a guinea pig.** For an upscale salon haircut without the upscale price, book an appointment for one of the salon's training nights. You'll pay little-to-no-money for a junior stylist to trim your tresses—usually with one of the head honchos standing by to protect you against any mistakes.

**Buy makeup during bonus time.** If you want to splurge on department store makeup, at least wait until they're giving away those fun goodie bags. Most contain a mini-mascara, lipstick, and tube of moisturizing cream that could last you for months.

**Know when to cheap out.** No need to pay through the nose for a super-hip eye shadow you'll be sick of in a week. Drugstores, dollar emporiums, and trendy clothing stores such as H&M are great spots to find the hottest styles—without breaking the bank.

**Share your clothes.** How to double your wardrobe without spending a penny? Team up with any friends who share your size (and taste) in fashion, and hold a clothing swap.

# your crowning moment

## Amelia Vega, Dominican Republic, Miss Universe 2003

As the Miss Universe 2003 competition drew to a nail-biting close, Amelia Vega stood on a stage in Panama City, Panama, clasping hands with Miss Venezuela (Mariangel Ruiz Torrealba) and waiting to hear who would go home with the title. Her mind racing, Amelia caught the eyes of her friends and family in the audience. She spotted groups of strangers—many carrying flags from other countries—who enthusiastically cheered her on. And then she prayed—hard. "I said, 'God, if you think I'm not ready to handle this big responsibility, don't give it to me,'" Amelia recalls. "And then they called my name as Miss Universe."

She had spent nearly a year working hard for this day, taking classes in oratory, poise, and even the art of gliding gracefully down a catwalk. Always in the front of her mind was the driving knowledge that no one from the Dominican Republic had ever won the Miss Universe crown. Yet nothing could truly prepare Amelia for the moment her name was called. "You can watch it now on the video—the first thing I did was look up, cross my chest, and whisper 'Thank you,'" she says. "Then I thought, 'Now what? I have a whole year ahead of me. This is only the first step.'"

Right this minute, women of all ages, from all walks of life and from all cultures, are having crowning moments of their own. Perhaps one has just landed a plum job interview and is preparing for her chance to shine. Maybe another is stepping up to the marriage altar gleaming in head-to-toe white. Every woman encounters times like these—when the most important eyes in the room are focused directly on her. It's precisely during those times that we could all learn a little something from Miss Universe.

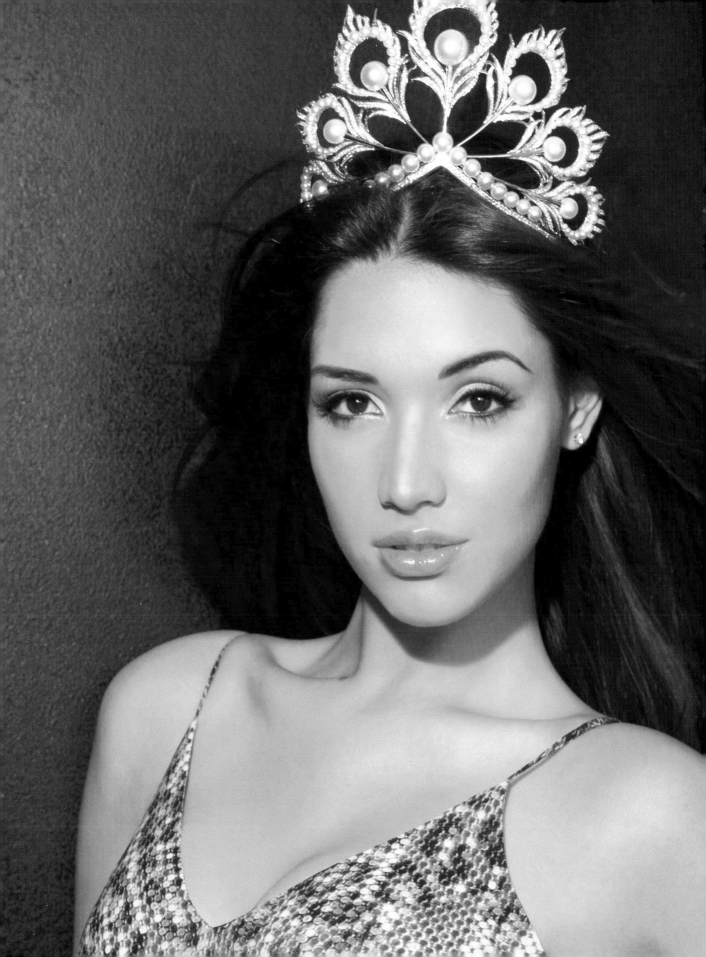

# clothes make the woman

Your moment in the spotlight really is just that—a moment. Experts say that it takes just a few short seconds to make a first impression. A few seconds to make or break that job interview, win over the crowd at that fabulous cocktail party, or ace an office presentation. Which means, like it or not, the clothes you choose to wear on these momentous occasions are everything. The trick, however, is looking beyond clothes that are simply fashionable—and selecting ones that truly flatter your body. Who cares if a pair of jeans looked hot on a runway model if it doesn't look hot on you? As the stylist for Miss Universe, Miss USA, and Miss Teen USA, Billie Causieestko is charged with making women of all different shapes and sizes look amazing on a daily basis—whether they're sipping champagne at a club in New York or addressing a roomful of ambassadors at the United Nations. Now, she shares a bit of her wisdom with us.

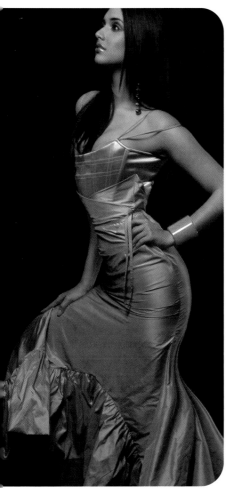

Amelia Vega, Dominican Republic, Miss Universe 2003

## the tall girl's shopping list

Men's trousers. They look great paired with a fitted, feminine top, a string of pearls, and strappy sandals.

Long gowns. Look for one with flowing fabric that swings around your long legs. For an especially dramatic formal look, try a dress with a short train.

An empire waist. For those who are low on curves, it can add the illusion of fuller breasts and hips.

Accessories. Though you don't want to pile it on, longer bodies can get away with more jewelry, belts, and bags. A belted monochromatic suit is an especially flattering look.

WATCH OUT FOR . . . Very short skirts, which can look cheap and scream "teenybopper" on long legs.

## the shorter girl's shopping list

Slim pants and skinny jeans. They elongate the legs, especial-ly when paired with a great pair of heels and a tunic on top.

High-waisted pencil skirts. Particularly great for less curvy types, they make your lower half look lean and long.

Skirts with front or side slits. This cocktail party favorite makes legs look longer by showing them off.

**Deep, V-necked tops.** Besides being a sexy option for evening, they direct the eyes downward, creating the illusion of a longer torso.

**A long chain necklace.** Worn as the centerpiece of your outfit, it helps lengthen the torso.

**WATCH OUT FOR . . .** Too many accessories. Piling on the bags and baubles can overwhelm a petite body.

## the ruler-shaped girl's shopping list

**Wide-legged pants with a corseted top or cinched jacket.** This classic pair fakes an hourglass shape.

**Slim, high-waisted skirts.** Whether worn at the office or at an evening event, they create the impression of rounder hips.

**Sleek mules.** Sexy heels make straight legs look a little more shapely.

**Jersey knits.** Fabric that drapes easily over the body accentuates subtle curves.

**Bias-cut skirts and dresses.** Asymmetry lends shape to a sleek physique.

**Plunging necklines.** They look beautiful—not vulgar—on those without a lot on top.

**WATCH OUT FOR . . .** Oversized clothes or boxy tops and jackets.

## the curvy girl's shopping list

**Well-tailored suits.** Clothes with a structured silhouette emphasize the body's natural shape.

**Trumpet skirts.** Provided you're not very round at the belly, skirts that are fitted at the hips and thighs—and flare out at the bottom—elongate the torso, drop the waist, and flatter your curves.

**A cinched jacket.** Tops that hug your middle show off your hourglass shape, as long as they don't amp up your cleavage too much.

**WATCH OUT FOR . . .** Tops that are too revealing. If you think you're putting on too much of a peep show, you probably are.

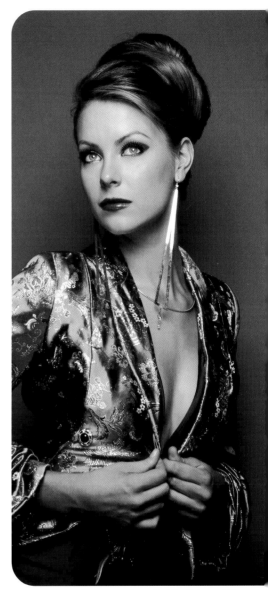

Jennifer Hawkins, Australia, Miss Universe 2004

# accessories: the icing on the cake

Before jetting off to Bangkok to compete for the crown, Natalie Glebova (Canada, Miss Universe 2005) visited a jewelry designer back home. "I brought in a lot of the outfits I was planning to wear while I was away," she recalls. "They custom-made one set of accessories for every outfit. It's amazing how you can wear an ordinary simple top, throw on a necklace—all of a sudden, it looks like so much more." The days when handbags, scarves, and jewelry were considered optional extras are over. "We are totally in an accessories-driven market right now," says Causieestko. "They're such a great way to add an instant, individual style to otherwise basic clothes. But there's definitely an artistic way of wearing them. Overkill really can kill your whole look."

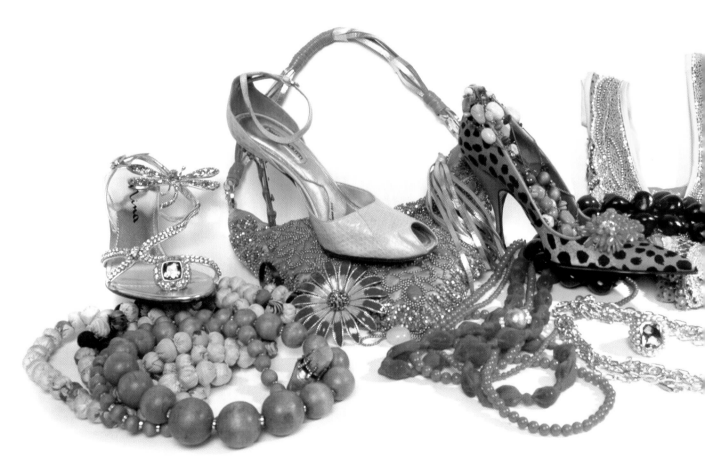

# universal truth

Color, when worn well, can make an outfit just as well as any accessory. So it behooves you to determine which shades flatter you best—and stick with them. When someone compliments you on an outfit, take note of what color you're wearing—or just look in your closet. "Most of us gravitate toward our best colors when we're shopping for clothes," says Causieestko. But if you're still stuck on which hue is you, consider these guidelines: Black looks amazing on olive-skinned brunettes, white looks right on women with darker complexions, and blues and turquoises are perfect for blondes with fair skin.

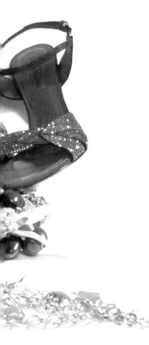

Don't play matchmaker. Matching your shoes with your bag is no longer necessary—and can even look a little passé, warns Causieestko. "I think one of the biggest fashion crimes is to wear a gold shoe with a gold handbag," she says. Instead, pair those shoes with a cute floral bag.

And speaking of gold. Metallics are huge right now—and they show no sign of going away. Gold shoes, a silver evening bag, and a sequined halter top all look fabulous—just not together. Choose one shiny accessory, then give it center stage.

Keep the background simple. Even if you're not doing metallic, it's important to maintain a sense of balance when accessorizing. While a handful of women can pull off pairing a funky outfit with equally funky extras, the rest of us are better off keeping one of those elements simple. "It's very tricky to be Madonna or Bjork," says Causieestko. "Instead, think of Sarah Jessica Parker in those Gap ads. A basic, fitted T and a pair of jeans are perfect with a great rhinestone belt and a pair of slingbacks."

Work it. Accessories are generally acceptable in even the most corporate offices—as long as you wear them judiciously. A good rule of thumb is to choose only functional items: watches, belts, and handbags. Keep those pared down and sophisticated, then consider adding one more nonfunctional extra, like a string of pearls, a brooch, or (if you work in a more creative field) a necklace with a quirky pendant. "Scarves also work really well, if you want to add some color," says Causieestko. "They're sort of the counterpart to a guy's tie."

Then play. Dashing from cubicle to cocktail fête is easy if you tuck the right finishing touches into your bag. A sparkly scarf, chandelier earrings, or a pair of strappy stilettos can turn a plain scoop-necked black shift into a festive party dress. Add a slim evening purse and you're good to go!

# how to look graceful in heels

Aside from the sash and crown, the mark of a genuine Miss Universe boils down to one question: How does she do in heels? Natalie Glebova does quite well, thank you very much. Before winning her title, she glided across the stage in four-inch stilettos as the hem of her evening gown swirled precariously around her feet. Meanwhile, the millions of women watching at home were eyeing Natalie's feet with a combination of awe and envy, asking, "How does she do it?" No doubt, a fabulous pair of heels can make a ho-hum set of legs look longer, leaner, and more elegant—assuming, that is, you know how to wear them.

Find comfortable shoes. It doesn't matter how low or high the heel is—if they don't fit properly, you'll be a hobbling mess. Rather than going for the skyscraper-high heels, consider a two-inch lift—you'll still get height and will wreak far less havoc on your feet. And be sure to take several laps around the shoe store—preferably on uncarpeted ground—before purchasing the shoes.

Take test drives. The key to looking like you live in heels? "Practice," says Natalie, who had logged many, many hours in her stilettos before prancing around the Miss Universe stage. Wearing your heels around the house for half an hour a day will not only help you get used to them, but also break them in so that you're less likely to get blisters later on.

Get the walk down. With your toes pointing straight ahead (not out to the sides) and your legs close together, step on your heel, rolling smoothly onto the ball of your foot. To keep your balance, swing your arms as you walk. And keep your eyes peeled for uneven surfaces where your pointed heels might sink or catch.

Then add the evening gown. Natalie's secret for high-heeling it in an evening gown: Kick each leg at the knee. "You want to kick the fabric away from your shoes with each step," she says. "If the dress is long, no one will be able to tell you're kicking."

Keep calm during calamities. If your skirt or dress catches a heel, stop and "continue to kick your foot very subtly until you untangle yourself," says Natalie. "Above all, you don't want your face to look like something has gone wrong. Smiling always works wonders."

Take them off. Again, the higher the heel, the more your feet suffer—both short term and long term. To save your tootsies, slip off your heels under your office desk, between meetings, on the way to a cocktail party, and whenever possible.

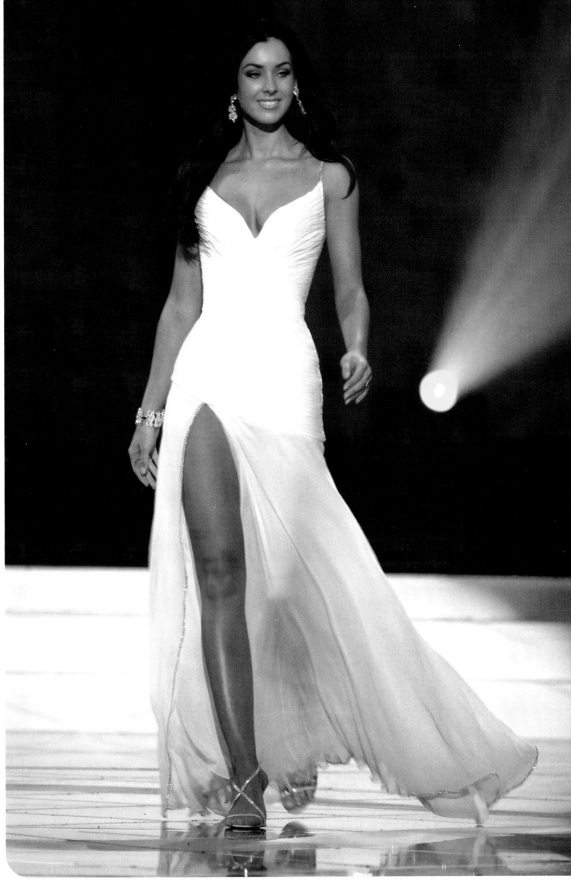

Natalie Glebova, Canada, Miss Universe 2005

# poise, please

A slim pencil skirt and the perfect pair of mules will definitely help you shine brighter when all eyes are on you. But as Natalie Glebova proved during her crowning moment, the best accessory of all is one you can't buy in any store. We're talking about poise—that elusive quality that's part charm, part grace, and part something utterly undefinable. Sylvia Hitchcock Carson (USA, Miss Universe 1967) sums it up best when she speculates on why she won the crown: "A cameraman told me it was because of the way my rear end looked when I walked, others said it was because of my radiance. I thought it was because I came across as being genuine and sincere." Do pageant winners have poise written into their DNA? Do they have a secret rule book the rest of us don't? Perhaps it's a little bit of both.

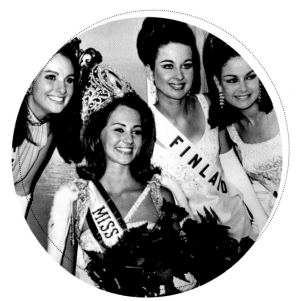

Sylvia Hitchcock Carson, USA, Miss Universe 1967

## universal truth

Big presentation or speech coming up? Steal a trick from Sylvia Hitchcock Carson. Here's how she keeps her smile looking fresh and engaging on stage: "When you're up there in front of a huge audience, find someone who isn't smiling and aim to make that person grin. You'll just radiate."

Use your eyes. Model Heidi Albertsen, who judged the Miss Universe competition in 2005, notes that carrying yourself well starts with good eye contact. "We judges were told to look at the eyes, but it applies in everyday life, too. There's nothing worse than when someone looks in the other direction when she's talking to you. It makes you feel like she's not really interested. Eyes really do speak louder than words." That said, Albertsen warns that eye contact isn't synonymous with staring. You want to look engaged and lively, not zombie-like.

Smile like you mean it. Jitters are normal when you're the center of attention. But the frowning and fidgeting that accompanies them can be a definite image breaker. Albertsen's simple solution: "Smile and the world will smile back. It's just about the friendliest thing you can do and the easiest way to give your face a natural radiance." And because the act of grinning increases the body's level of endorphins, you'll feel lighter and, yes, less jittery instantly.

Say hello. It sounds like a no-brainer, but people need reminding. Whether you're meeting a client for lunch or attending a big wedding reception, remember that you're not the only one who feels bashful. Taking the initiative with a handshake and engaging introduction immediately puts your companions at ease—and you come off glowing like the Hope Diamond.

Let your body talk. Your mannerisms and gestures are so ingrained, you probably don't even notice them— but others do. Crossing your arms or folding them over your chest tells your audience that you're closed off and guarded. Shifting your crossed legs away from the person you're talking to signals a lack of interest. Reprogramming yourself to speak more positive body language isn't hard—just start paying attention to your gestures and ask good friends to gently nudge you in the right direction.

Pause for some reflection. 1967 crown-winner Sylvia Hitchcock Carson, who now teaches seminars on image and presentation, says that many pageant winners are experts in the art of mirroring. "Figure out what's important to your audience and reflect it back to them," she says. "If you think about it, we're attracted to people who think like us."

Read the papers. In fact, read anything you can get your hands on and you'll always have a ready supply of fresh icebreakers. "Knowing what's happening in the news is crucial to carrying on lively conversation in any setting," says Albertsen, who believes that celebrity gossip magazines are also required reading. After all, you could walk into a party not knowing a soul—as long as you know who's dating who in Hollywood, you'll have plenty of gab partners.

Do some good. Ever notice how some of the most polished, graceful women in the world also happen to have big, generous hearts? After taking home the crown and having a commemorative postal stamp created in her honor, Denise M. Quiñones August (Puerto Rico, Miss Universe 2001) has continued to give back. Her tireless work against HIV/AIDS has been recognized by both the Centers for Disease Control and the American Foundation for AIDS Research.

# how to wow anyone you meet

Brook Lee (USA, Miss Universe 1997) knows how to work a room. During her reign and in the years since, she's charmed everyone from prime ministers to flight attendants. We coaxed her to reveal a few of her secrets.

Dazzle your future boss. Always arrive at a job interview fifteen minutes early, and enter with a smile. Remember that you're the one who has something to offer them—if you weren't fully qualified for the job, you wouldn't be there. Remember that most of the time, personality bears more weight than the credentials on your resume. It's your people skills—whether or not you're a pleasant person to be around—that employers tend to notice first. As for appearance, never, ever wear anything you wouldn't feel comfortable wearing around your parents or people you respect. A job interview is not a time to experiment with a new look. Keep in mind that it's hardly a crime to be overdressed—but it's always a mark against you if you look too casual. This sends the signal that you have no respect for yourself or for the spot you're interviewing for.

Make an entrance at a splashy party. Mingle, mingle, mingle! If you know a lot of people there, resist the urge to plant yourself in one tiny circle of friends. Instead, be a moving target. When you do approach someone new, you might start by asking her where she got her bag or how she knows the hostess. There is no reason to delve into serious issues when everyone's making small talk. Keep it light.

Get a stranger to take you seriously. A firm handshake is a must. "I can't tell you how many dignitaries and heads of state I have met who were surprised that I had such a firm handshake," says Brook. "My father taught me early that people will judge your character from your handshake." Especially if you are a woman, a firm handshake says you are confident, competent, and not someone that needs to be handled with kid gloves.

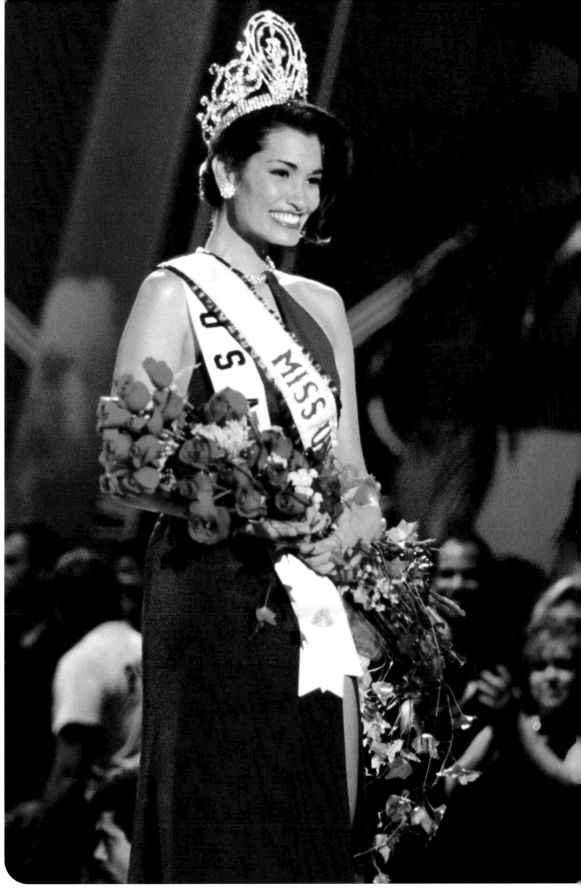

Brook Lee, USA, Miss Universe 1997

# this magic moment

The road to Miss Universe is a long, bumpy one. It's a journey filled with struggles, tears, laughter, and joy. Here is a look at a few of our favorite crowning moments, along with reflections from past winners on their trips to the top.

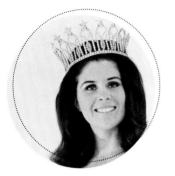

"I went to the Miss USA pageant with a borrowed bright yellow empire-waist bridesmaid's dress, with no low-cut neck. I used to be the head majorette at my high school, and to me, being in the pageant was like performing. I loved being there with all the girls."

—Sylvia Hitchcock Carson, USA, Miss Universe 1967

"I was not really beautiful when I was a little girl. There were pageants in my school, but I never won anything—I wasn't even invited to be in them. But when I was twelve, I grew boobs and grew tall. When I turned fourteen, people started asking me to do pageants."

—Martha Vasconcellos, Brazil, Miss Universe 1968

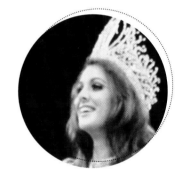

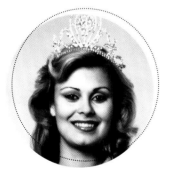

"The excitement grew as each runner-up was announced. Finally, Miss Haiti and I were standing there holding hands. She was so beautiful and lovely, and I was almost sure that she would win. When the result was announced, I remember the cheers and applause of the audience—and walking to the throne exhilarated and feeling like a queen."

—Anne Marie Pohtamo, Finland, Miss Universe 1975

"When I was a little girl, I always liked to dress nicely, maybe because of the influence of my mother. She had been a contestant in the Miss Madrid pageant; I think she came in third or fourth place. I always saw her taking care of herself and putting on makeup."

—Maritza Sayalero, Venezuela, Miss Universe 1979

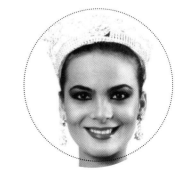

## 8. When in your life have you felt most beautiful?

Giving birth to my three children.

## 9. How do you define beauty?

Beauty radiates from within and is only appreciated when shared with others.

## 10. What person—living or dead—represents true beauty to you?

Jesus, because spirituality and beauty go hand and hand.

## 11. Which souvenirs have you kept from your Miss Universe experience? Which item(s) mean the most to you?

Photographs and articles documenting my experience during my reign as Miss Alabama, Miss USA, and Miss Universe—especially one photo taken on stage with my parents and brother Ralph, who had returned from the Vietnam War.

## 12. What is your best memory of the Miss Universe Pageant?

Actually winning and feeling the pride I brought my parents, family, and supportive friends. Also, exploring the cultures of other contestants.

## 13. If you could change one thing about the day you won the crown, what would it be?

Nothing—it was perfect!

## 14. What's your best beauty secret?

Smiling, having a positive attitude, plus thinking young!

## 15. What's the best piece of beauty advice you've ever been given? Who gave you this advice?

To your own self be true—from my own namesake, Aunt Sylvia Little, of North Andover, Massachusetts.

# Martha Vasconcellos, Brazil
# Miss Universe 1968

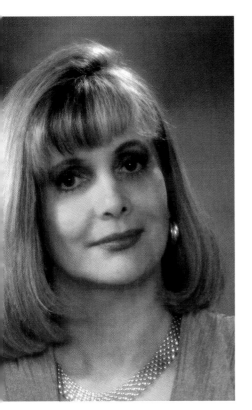

1. When is the first time you remember wearing makeup?

   When I was fifteen. Before that, I wasn't allowed to wear it.

2. How often do you wear it now?

   I wear it every day, even when I'm at home. If my boyfriend, John, is around, I always have it on.

3. Who do you wear makeup for?

   I really feel better when I wear makeup, because I feel very pale when I don't. I wear it for myself.

4. If you were stranded on a desert island, which single beauty product would you choose to have with you? Why?

   Floss and a toothbrush. When I don't floss after eating, I feel as if I'm wearing a tight shoe.

5. What is your favorite beauty ritual?

   Getting into a Jacuzzi. I have candles and oils, and a special loofah. When I lived in Brazil, I took one every day after going to the gym.

6. Which is your least favorite and why?

   Shaving.

7. What is in your shower caddy right now?

   Shampoo, conditioner, body wash, facial soap, a sponge, and a pumice stone.

8. When in your life have you felt most beautiful?

   I feel the most beautiful when I'm in love with someone—that means my heart is having a ball.

9. How do you define beauty?

Internal peace.

10. What person—living or dead—represents true beauty to you?

My father—he was a very handsome man.

11. Which souvenirs have you kept from your Miss Universe experience? Which item(s) mean the most to you?

I have the trophy, all the magazines, newspapers, many pictures. I still have my dress and bathing suit—everything. The trophy is what means the most. Because at the time, we weren't allowed to keep the crown.

12. What is your best memory of the Miss Universe Pageant?

It's not my best, but the day I won, I was not really happy. I was afraid. My father didn't like the idea that I was in a beauty pageant. After I won, I couldn't even answer any of the questions they were asking me backstage. People thought I was crying because I was happy. I was crying because I was worried.

13. If you could change one thing about the day you won the crown, what would it be?

I wish my father had been more receptive. I came from a very conservative family that belonged to the social elite. If I had won an award for, say, academic excellence, he would have been very proud, but a beauty pageant? That was something else! My father had real misgivings about that kind of public exposure.

14. What's your best beauty secret?

If I tell you, it's not a secret anymore.

15. What's the best piece of beauty advice you've ever been given? Who gave you this advice?

When I was fifteen, my mother put me into a class at the local women's club. They taught me how to be a lady. One of the teachers taught me everything about how to behave, how to walk, how to have nice posture, and how to wear makeup. This course was important for the rest of my life.

# Margaret Gardiner, South Africa
# Miss Universe 1978

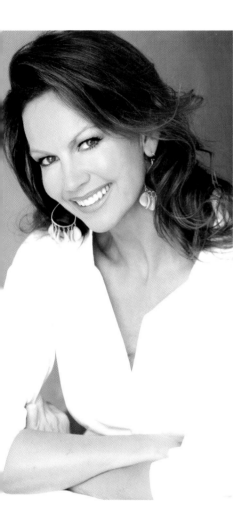

1. ## When is the first time you remember wearing makeup?

   Lip gloss at age thirteen.

2. ## How often do you wear it now?

   As a professional television journalist I have to wear it often. When I'm home I go naked-skinned. When running around town I use lipstick. Even if nothing else is there the color brings out the eyes.

3. ## Who do you wear makeup for?

   Unless I'm in a professional situation where there are expectations, I wear it for myself. My opinion of myself is more important than anyone else's. Makeup can lift me on a bad day, but is totally useless when camping.

4. ## If you were stranded on a desert island, which single beauty product would you choose to have with you. Why?

   Mascara. I used to be white blonde as a kid and although my hair changed, my skin stayed horribly white. Mascara creates contrast at the eyes and can be twirled over the eyebrows. But if I were on a desert island, I wouldn't care what I looked like! I may be a beauty queen, but I'm not stupid.

5. ## What is your favorite beauty ritual?

   Soaking in a tub.

6. ## Which is your least favorite and why?

   Sunscreen. But in L.A., where the sun is constant and you get fried in a car speeding around town, it's just necessary—and laborious.

7. ## What is in your shower caddy right now?

   Loofah, loofah, loofah! And butter body cream.

8. ## When in your life have you felt most beautiful?

   We all have power days, when somehow we look right, but I feel best after a good workout. I feel most beautiful when I'm with my son. Unconditional love will do that to you.

## 9. How do you define beauty?

I've met some ugly people who are beautiful and the other way around. Many movie stars, who I see on a daily basis as part of my job, are not beautiful—or at least not the most beautiful. But through the way they carry themselves and a combination of personality, confidence, and making the best of what they've got, they become the most beautiful. There is a scary thing happening in L.A. All the women are having work done to take away the traits that make them individuals. There is a sameness to the look that is unnatural. It is the opposite of beauty.

## 10. What person—living or dead—represents true beauty to you?

Any child. Have you looked at children when they are playing? Happiness is unfiltered and it makes them stunning. Each one of them. I've also had the pleasure of meeting some of the great beauties of our day—and the down side of being photographed with them! Sophia Loren was stunning.

## 11. Which souvenirs have you kept from your Miss Universe experience? Which item(s) mean the most to you?

For years my crown was kept in my garage in Africa where my mum lives. She has everything. If you walked into my home you would not be able to tell that I had won the title. There is nothing to the casual observer. But in my kitchen is a tiny figurine that I received while competing in the Miss Universe Pageant. I don't notice it every day, but when I see it, it reminds me of a time more than twenty years ago, when I was a different person.

## 12. What is your best memory of the Miss Universe Pageant?

Other than winning, the cultures I got exposed to and the girls. When else can you get together with representatives from the rest of the world and explore friendships? Miss Trinidad & Tobago and I used to sit at the back of the bus singing songs with a group of other contestants. Miss Australia and I bought a drink and watched the sun set over the white beaches of Mexico. Visiting Chichén Itzá was a highlight—and the Mexican people were fantastic.

## 13. If you could change one thing about the day you won the crown, what would it be?

I'd slow it down so I could remember it better.

## 14. What's your best beauty secret?

Rest.

## 15. What's the best piece of beauty advice you've ever been given? Who gave you this advice?

It's something I learned modeling internationally and traveling as Miss Universe. Sleep whenever you can. Because of all the time zones and the need to be polite and friendly in public, the grueling hours I worked then prepared me for life in general. The rules a public personality has to absorb are the ones that help you in life.
Be calm. Think before you talk. Sleep whenever you can. Conserve your energy. Be nice.

# Maritza Sayalero, Venezuela
# Miss Universe 1979

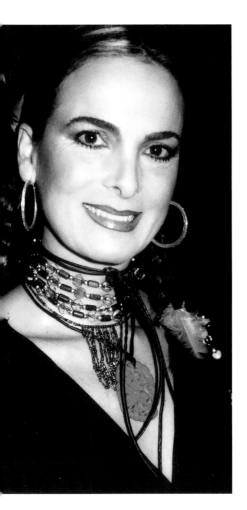

1.  **When is the first time you remember wearing makeup?**

    My first memory of that is on the day of my fifteenth birthday.

2.  **How often do you wear it now?**

    Very often, but it depends on the occasion.

3.  **Who do you wear makeup for?**

    First for me to feel and look good—and then for others.

4.  **If you were stranded on a desert island, which single beauty product would you choose to have with you? Why?**

    A facial exfoliation gel would be nice because I like my face to look healthy and rejuvenated.

5.  **What is your favorite beauty ritual?**

    Getting a good facial and having my eyebrows done by my daughter—she's an aesthetician.

6.  **Which is your least favorite and why?**

    Doing my hair, because it takes too long to get it the way I like.

7.  **What is in your shower caddy right now?**

    Shampoo, conditioner, a sponge, and body exfoliator.

8.  **When in your life have you felt most beautiful?**

    The day I won Miss Universe, the day I got married, and the day I gave birth.

9. How do you define beauty?

A combination of physical looks and inner strength.

10. What person—living or dead—represents true beauty to you?

My mother gets my vote.

11. Which souvenirs have you kept from your Miss Universe experience? Which item(s) mean the most to you?

Many souvenirs are very special: my crown, my trophy, and my sash.

12. What is your best memory of the Miss Universe Pageant?

The moment they called my name: "Maritza Sayalero, Miss Universe."

13. If you could change one thing about the day you won the crown, what would it be?

I'd keep the stage from falling down. [A rush of reporters and contestants caused the stage to collapse after Maritza was crowned.]

14. What's your best beauty secret?

No secret—eat right, exercise, and stay happy.

15. What's the best piece of beauty advice you've ever been given? Who gave you this advice?

For sure, exercise makes my body and mind feel good. (My husband.)

# Porntip "Bui" Nakhirunkanok Simon, Thailand, Miss Universe 1988

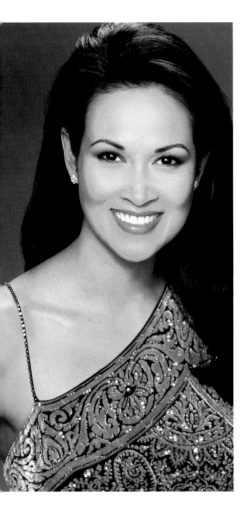

1. **When is the first time you remember wearing makeup?**

   I was sixteen. My mom was strict. She didn't want us growing up too fast. I'd sneak my mascara and lipstick to school and arrive half an hour early to put it on.

2. **How often do you wear it now?**

   I can do with just a little blush and lipstick every day. I try to go at least two days a week without makeup to let my skin breathe.

3. **Who do you wear makeup for?**

   My husband and I do a lot of entertaining at home.

4. **If you were stranded on a desert island, which single beauty product would you choose to have with you? Why?**

   My sunblock—I don't want to get burned.

5. **What is your favorite beauty ritual?**

   My nighttime treatment. After I take a bath, I apply all my potions and lotions, and I feel really taken care of.

6. **Which is your least favorite and why?**

   Putting on makeup. It just seems so repetitive. Even my daughter thinks so. She'll ask, "You're painting your face again?"

7. **What is in your shower caddy right now?**

   Shampoo, face scrub, body scrub, conditioner, and a comb.

8. **When in your life have you felt most beautiful?**

   When I was pregnant. For some reason, I got more compliments than I ever did in my life. Men, especially, would stop me on the street and tell me how beautiful I was. When you're pregnant, you don't bother fussing with makeup. It just goes to show, you can fuss all day, but natural beauty screams louder.

## 9. How do you define beauty?

Beauty starts with the person. If you're not going to take care of yourself and honor yourself and appreciate yourself, how can somebody else? Beauty starts with liking who you are. That affects how you care for your hair, wear your clothes, and so on.

## 10. What person—living or dead—represents true beauty to you?

Audrey Hepburn. I adore that woman. I had the privilege of meeting her once. She was the epitome of grace and beauty—minimal makeup, hair pulled back, very tailored suits, nothing flashy. Her beauty came from who she is. There was such confidence about her.

## 11. Which souvenirs have you kept from your Miss Universe experience? Which item(s) mean the most to you?

The best is the crown. I keep it in my office—that's my private space. It's nice to know that I share that crown with only a few dozen women in history. And my photographs from that year, showing my travels, the presidents I've met, the accomplishments that I've made.

## 12. What is your best memory of the Miss Universe Pageant?

Nothing can compare with having that crown slammed on your head. Then, as soon as you go off the air, all the photographers come up on stage. You feel like Dorothy in *The Wizard of Oz*.

## 13. If you could change one thing about the day you won the crown, what would it be?

Obviously, everything went right for me. I got to stand where I did. To change anything would be superficial at this point.

## 14. What's your best beauty secret?

Rest. I think women in particular need rest. We use so much energy in our day and I think rest is such an underestimated necessity. People think they need to do more, and in doing so we let down our bodies. I don't get sick; when I feel my body is on overload, I go to bed an extra hour early to let my body recharge. I think that helps keep away wrinkles, irritability, fatigue, and sickness.

## 15. What's the best piece of beauty advice you've ever been given? Who gave you this advice?

When I was sixteen, I got a gift certificate to a beauty spa for a facial. That really was the best secret I could've been given. I met this woman named Vera Brown who taught me all about skin care. Because of her, I never had to have pimples. She taught me at an early age how to respect skin: Don't stay out in the sun, don't go to bed with a dirty face, keep your skin in balance.

# Angela Visser, Holland
# Miss Universe 1989

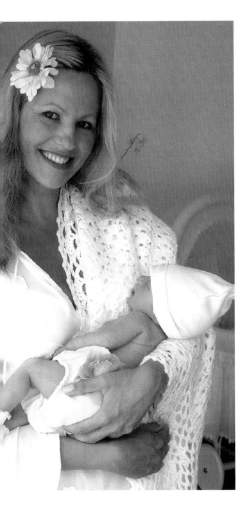

1. ## When is the first time you remember wearing makeup?

   During a ballet recital when I was a little girl, probably around five years old. I remember it being really exciting, wearing the tutu and the fake eyelashes! I didn't really start to wear makeup until I was a teenager, and then only once in a while.

2. ## How often do you wear it now?

   Almost on a daily basis. The amount or what depends on the occasion.

3. ## Who do you wear makeup for?

   For myself.

4. ## If you were stranded on a desert island, which single beauty product would you choose to have with you? Why?

   Moisturizing cream with SPF. I could use it on my face, my lips, my body, my nails, and my feet, and keep my hair back with it!

5. ## What is your favorite beauty ritual?

   Taking a morning shower with my little baby, Amelie.

6. ## Which is your least favorite and why?

   I don't have a least favorite ritual. If I didn't like it, I wouldn't make it a ritual.

7. ## What is in your shower caddy right now?

   A rubber ducky; a rubber octopus; a rubber frog; Mustela baby hair and body wash; Kiehl's scrub; Neutrogena shampoo, conditioner, and shower gel; a razor; and shaving cream.

## 8. When in your life have you felt most beautiful?

After giving birth to baby Amelie—the moment where they put her on my stomach and we looked at each other for the first time. Nothing can compare to that moment—I have never felt more happy or beautiful!

## 9. How do you define beauty?

A happy, loving, radiant spirit.

## 10. What person—living or dead—represents true beauty to you?

My mother. She is my inspiration in life.

## 11. Which souvenirs have you kept from your Miss Universe experience? Which item(s) mean the most to you?

Everything! Besides, of course, the crown, everything means a lot because it was given or handmade by people all over the world, who I did not know and who were so nice and generous. I could never not keep all those things! Another thing that means a lot to me is my handprints on the Walk of Fame in Holland. I feel very honored that I am part of that incredible group of people.

## 12. What is your best memory of the Miss Universe Pageant?

Seeing my parents' and my brother's faces after I had won—their smiles and the little Dutch flag they were waving. They were three little dots in an audience of many, but seeing them and knowing they had experienced this with me meant everything!

## 13. If you could change one thing about the day you won the crown, what would it be?

Nothing—it was a perfect day.

## 14. What's your best beauty secret?

Love and be loved.

## 15. What's the best piece of beauty advice you've ever been given? Who gave you this advice?

Always keep smiling! My mother.

# Brook Lee, USA
## Miss Universe 1997

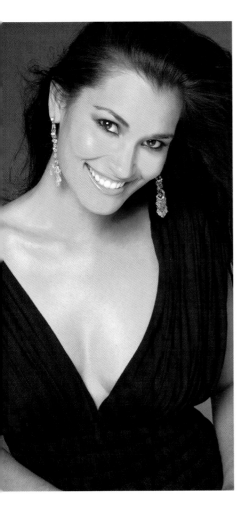

1. When is the first time you remember wearing makeup?

   I was very little, but it was only for the stage. I have been dancing hula since I was two years old.

2. How often do you wear it now?

   I only wear it for work or auditions, and an occasional night out. Otherwise, I like to let my skin breathe.

3. Who do you wear makeup for?

   Predominantly for work and to go out. But I always tend to feel when I put makeup on that I am "working."

4. If you were stranded on a desert island, which single beauty product would you choose to have with you? Why?

   Sunscreen! Okay, and lip balm. I would imagine it would be sunny on an island, and if it's deserted who do I really have to look good for? Plus, the longer I can preserve my skin, the "younger" I can look when those hot sailors come to the rescue.

5. What is your favorite beauty ritual?

   I love doing masks, either at home or a spa. It forces me to slow down and take it easy because I can't go anywhere or really multitask with goop on my face.

6. Which is your least favorite and why?

   I don't really care for manicures and pedicures—they are tedious. I always end up nicking a nail—it's annoying.

7. What is in your shower caddy right now?

   I don't have a caddy, but I do have the best Listchi soap. I got it as a gift and it's from a line called Fresh.

8. When in your life have you felt most beautiful?

Still working on that.

9. How do you define beauty?

I totally (and, yes, it's a cliché) believe it is from within. If you feel good about yourself, it shines through, how comfortable you are in your skin, how gracious you can be to others.

10. What person—living or dead—represents true beauty to you?

Another favorite cliché—but Audrey Hepburn. Without a doubt, the woman embraced every stage of her life from ingénue to death with such serenity and total grace. She is timeless, classic, and a truly beautiful being inside and out.

11. Which souvenirs have you kept from your Miss Universe experience? Which item(s) mean the most to you?

I have a ton of stuff from my year. If there is one thing you can count on besides the crown, it is all the stuff people give you from all over the world. It is hard to pick one thing. I guess the weirdest would be a rock from the DMZ in Korea. My father served after the war, and being Korean, it's kind of cool to know it's half North Korea, half South Korea.

12. What is your best memory of the Miss Universe Pageant?

I have so many great memories of my year as Miss Universe. But to be honest, the memories that really and truly stick with me are my days in the Miss Universe office hanging out with everybody, and how much fun it was to see it all come together.

13. If you could change one thing about the day you won the crown, what would it be?

I wouldn't change one thing. I had my family there, I had my friends there, I had the office there. It was a surprise for us all but it was so much fun.

14. What's your best beauty secret?

Sleep a lot—get as much sleep as you can—it helps preserve you longer!

15. What's the best piece of beauty advice you've ever been given? Who gave you this advice?

This girl I admired in grade school choir who was most popular, most talented, most liked, once told a bunch of us girls, always clean your face with Sea Breeze to unclog your pores. I don't use Sea Breeze, but I do wash my face every day and never, never go to bed with makeup on.

# Wendy Fitzwilliam, Trinidad & Tobago
# Miss Universe 1998

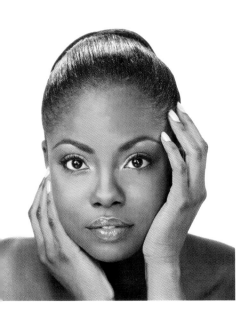

1. When is the first time you remember wearing makeup?

   When I received the Sacrament of Confirmation—I was fifteen.

2. How often do you wear it now?

   Every weekday to work, and to any social function.

3. Who do you wear makeup for?

   Definitely myself first and a public that expects me to look like I did on May 12, 1998, forever.

4. If you were stranded on a desert island, which single beauty product would you choose to have with you? Why?

   Water, lots of it. It's great for your skin, absolutely necessary for survival, and if that island is not much more than a sandbar in the salty ocean, I would so need that water. If the island has its own source of clean fresh water, then a pretty shade of red lipstick, which always dresses up any face with very little effort.

5. What is your favorite beauty ritual?

   A day spent at the spa starting with a full body massage, then a facial followed by a mani/pedi.

6. Which is your least favorite and why?

   Plucking my "stray eyebrows." Mum never warned me about that particular feature of getting older.

7. What is in your shower caddy right now?

   Jencare facial scrub, moisturizing body wash, Jencare facial wash, and a pair of exfoliating body gloves.

## 8. When in your life have you felt most beautiful?

At the most unremarkable times, or when I'm in love or excited about a new project. I've found my state of mind directly affects my "glow," which everyone around me sees immediately. Even if no one else can identify why, when I feel secure and happy, it is immediately reflected in the way I look.

## 9. What person—living or dead—represents true beauty to you?

Audrey Hepburn.

## 10. Which souvenirs have you kept from your Miss Universe experience? Which item(s) mean the most to you?

Pictures with some of my fellow delegates, my crown and sash. I'm still in touch with a few of the women I met. Miss USA, Shawnae Jebbia, has become a good friend—we even vacation together.

## 11. What is your best memory of the Miss Universe Pageant?

Two memories tie for first place. First, the moment I won and every delegate rushed forward to congratulate me—totally unscripted and in sheer enthusiasm we messed up the end of the live telecast. Instead of being crowned, the shot of me winning is of a surprised Wendy with Miss Ghana swinging from my neck in excitement and all the other delegates trying to hug and kiss me. Meanwhile, Scott, the choreographer, and Brook Lee, Miss Universe 1997, were begging everyone to step back for a minute so I could be crowned and sashed to take my walk. Second, the morning after winning when I got up excited and all alone in my suite to find two of the Central American delegates outside my door writing a note wishing me well. That was a very special moment—not the kind that usually makes the news about pageants, but a very special moment.

## 12. If you could change one thing about the day you won the crown, what would it be?

The earrings I wore. I begged Peter, my buddy and stylist, to please let me wear smaller earrings more in keeping with my personality and fashion sense. He insisted on the big ones, which I wore, and they totally clashed with that big crown.

## 13. What's your best beauty secret?

Drink lots of water and keep a positive outlook on life always, even in great difficulty. Nothing ages you like unhappiness and negativity.

# Amelia Vega, Dominican Republic
# Miss Universe 2003

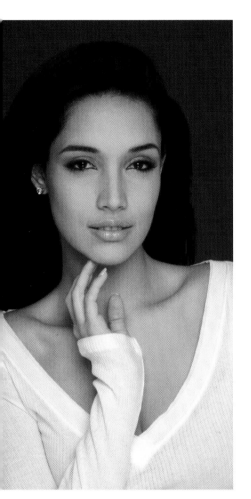

1. ## When is the first time you remember wearing makeup?

   When I was six years old, my grandmother told me she was going to Puerto Rico. She always liked to buy me things, so I told her I wanted beautiful heels, fake nails, and a lot of makeup! I've always been very girly—I always loved looking in the mirror and pretending I was a model or an actress or a singer.

2. ## How often do you wear it now?

   When I'm not working, I don't wear much. But makeup is still something I love to put on. Even when I run out to the pharmacy, I have to have something on my face.

3. ## Who do you wear makeup for?

   For myself. I want to look in the mirror and say, "Okay, I like how I look today."

4. ## If you were stranded on a desert island, which single beauty product would you choose to have with you? Why?

   Mascara—just think of pretty dolls and those huge eyelashes. I think eyes are very important. I could forget all my other makeup, but not mascara. I even wear it to the gym.

5. ## What is your favorite beauty ritual?

   Beauty sleep! You just don't look the same after you've been out to the clubs the night before. I try to get at least eight hours—more, if I can.

6. ## Which is your least favorite and why?

   Drinking water. It's hard to get into the habit, but it's so important. It gives the skin such a glow.

7. ## What is in your shower caddy right now?

   I've been out of my house for a month and a half traveling, but I always have my loofah. When I was a little girl, my grandmother would always tell me to use it on my elbows and knees. It makes my skin so soft.

## 8. When in your life have you felt most beautiful?

I think beauty changes with the years—and every stage of life has a certain beauty. I think I was a beautiful kid, but I could probably say I'm just as beautiful now. Beauty is about just being comfortable with yourself.

## 9. How do you define beauty?

It's different for everybody—but it's a combination of inner and outer beauty. The most important thing is to feel beautiful for yourself, not to make other people happy.

## 10. What person—living or dead—represents true beauty to you?

I can't really name one person. Everyone has a different kind of beauty, whether it's how you carry yourself or how gorgeous your face is.

## 11. Which souvenirs have you kept from your Miss Universe experience? Which item(s) mean the most to you?

I've kept all of them—I have a room full of boxes back home in the Dominican Republic with letters and pictures. I remember meeting a woman in a restaurant whose son had died in the World Trade Center. She had a bracelet inscribed with her son's name and an American flag. She said to me, "My son had your last name." Then she took off her bracelet and gave it to me.

## 12. What is your best memory of the Miss Universe Pageant?

It's impossible to name one. Every day was a different adventure with new faces and new countries. Knowing that thousands of people would come to a place just to see you—it was incredible.

## 13. If you could change one thing about the day you won the crown, what would it be?

I would have been able to see all the people I wanted to see. It all went by so fast.

## 14. What's your best beauty secret?

Have a good boyfriend! Also, I wear lotion to bed and take my makeup off every night, no matter how tired I am.

## 15. What's the best piece of beauty advice you've ever been given? Who gave you this advice?

Put egg whites on my face, let it dry, then rinse it off. The skin feels like a baby's afterwards.
My mom told me that one.

# Jennifer Hawkins, Australia
# Miss Universe 2004

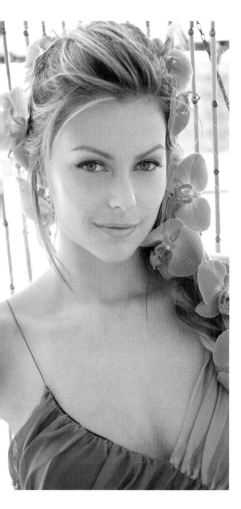

1. ## When is the first time you remember wearing makeup?

I was five, and it was my first ballet concert. I was allowed to wear bright red lipstick and a little blush—and I loved it.

2. ## How often do you wear it now?

At events and television appearances. Not too much, though. I like the fresh, bronze look.

3. ## Who do you wear makeup for?

I don't typically wear it, especially if I'm off to the beach. But if I'm working, I put on base, eye makeup, blush, and lip gloss. Otherwise, you'll look washed out on film. When I'm out dancing with my girlfriends or go out on a date, I'll wear some—it's fun to play around with different looks. But makeup is only good if it enhances beauty, not if it's covering everything up.

4. ## If you were stranded on a desert island, which single beauty product would you choose to have with you? Why?

Moisturizer—I can't go without it!

5. ## What is your favorite beauty ritual?

Washing my face, putting on a mask, moisturizing my whole body, and using eye cream.

6. ## Which is your least favorite and why?

Waxing.

7. ## What is in your shower caddy right now?

Lux body wash, face wash, and a loofah, and my toothbrush. I clean my teeth in the shower.

8.  When in your life have you felt most beautiful?

Whenever my mum and dad tell me I am—I know they mean it.

9.  How do you define beauty?

Confidence.

10.  What person—living or dead—represents true beauty to you?

That's a hard one—my list would go on and on.

11.  Which souvenirs have you kept from your Miss Universe experience? Which item(s) mean the most to you?

My contacts book—it has the list of the new friendships I've made along the way.

12.  What is your best memory of the Miss Universe Pageant?

The whole year. The travel, the different cultures, the events, the red carpet. Shopping and hanging out with my roommate, Chelsea Cooley (Miss USA 2005), in New York was pretty cool. The last night on stage—sooooo fun. So many things. I loved all of it.

13.  If you could change one thing about the day you won the crown, what would it be?

I wish I'd had family there. I told them not to come all the way to Ecuador, because I had no chance of winning. I was wrong.

14.  What's your best beauty secret?

I think water is the key to great skin.

15.  What's the best piece of beauty advice you've ever been given?

Less is sometimes more—don't overdo it.

# Natalie Glebova, Canada
# Miss Universe 2005

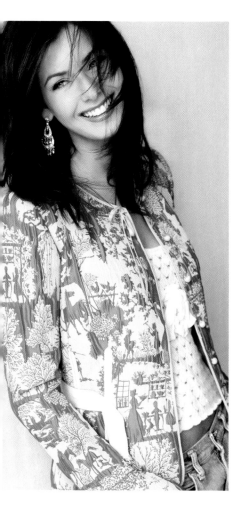

1. When is the first time you remember wearing makeup?

Fourteen years old.

2. How often do you wear it now?

Daily.

3. Who do you wear makeup for?

To go outside, especially when meeting other people.

4. If you were stranded on a desert island, which single beauty product would you choose to have with you? Why?

Moisturizing lotion. I love the feeling of smooth, silky skin. And I hate dry, flaky skin.

5. What is your favorite beauty ritual?

Applying makeup to go out. Especially glamorous makeup, the kind you can have fun and use your creativity with.

6. Which is your least favorite and why?

Painting my nails, because it takes a very long time. You have to sit still so you don't chip the nail polish. I always mess up at least one nail.

7. What is in your shower caddy right now?

Shampoo, conditioner, body wash, and body scrub.

8. When in your life have you felt most beautiful?

The first time that someone told me "I love you."

9. How do you define beauty?

Creative personal style, good grooming, and a great personality.

10. What person—living or dead—represents true beauty to you?

Elizabeth Taylor.

11. Which souvenirs have you kept from your Miss Universe experience? Which item(s) mean the most to you?

I've kept the book that has all of the contestants' pictures, and I had it signed by many of them. I keep it and read it from time to time; it always makes me smile.

12. What is your best memory of the Miss Universe Pageant?

Having our meals together at the hotel and rehearsal hall. Also, dancing and sharing stories from our countries with the girls.

13. If you could change one thing about the day you won the crown, what would it be?

I can't think of anything to change. It was a perfect moment, and everyone close to me was there to share it with me. I guess the only other people I wish were there are my grandparents.

14. What's your best beauty secret?

Self-tanner—it gives me a natural-looking tan without spending time (and damaging my skin) at the tanning salon. Bronzer also helps a lot.

15. What's the best piece of beauty advice you've ever been given? Who gave you this advice?

My mom always told me, "Sleep is the best beauty remedy." She's right! When I'm well rested I feel and look so much better.

# INDEX ●●●

## N

## O

Fadil Berisha Studios

Greg Harbaugh for Miss Universe L.P., LLLP

Darren Decker for Miss Universe L.P., LLLP

Patrick Prather for Miss Universe L.P., LLLP

Frank L. Szelwach for Miss Universe L.P., LLLP

Miss Universe L.P., LLLP Archives

Getty Images

Rick Day

Kimo Lauer

Mikimoto (America) Co., Ltd.

Farouk Systems, Inc.

Bachrach